100 WAYS TO KILL CANCER

Shuhua (Steve) Zheng, Ph.D.

Disclaimer

100 Ways to Kill Cancer aims at providing general principles and scientific discoveries of cancer research and its associated disciples. The book is NOT intended as a working guide to drug administration, patient care or treatment. It is the responsibility of the treating practioner to determine the best treatment and method of application for the patient. Neither the author nor the author and editor assume any liability for any injury and/or damage to the person or property arising from or related to the material within this publication.

Although care has be taken to issue the accuracy of information present in this publication, the author, editor and publisher make no representation or warranties whatsoever, express or implied, with respect to the completeness, accuracy or currency of the content of this publication. This publication is not meant to be a substitute for the advice of a physician or other licensed and qualified medical professionals. Information presented in this publication may refer to drugs, devices or techniques which are subject to government regulation, and it is the responsibility of the treating practioner to comply with all application laws.

To contact us, please email: 100waystokillcancer@gmail.com

Cover design is based on Canva Pty Ld. The authorization to use photocopy items in the book cover is granted under the license agreement of multi-use with no time limit.

Some artwork in the book is designed based on photocopy items published on www.pixabay.com. To the extent possible under law, images on Pixabay are released under Creative Commons CC0.

Copyright © 2018 Shuhua Zheng, Yue Meng

All rights reserved.

ISBN: 9781720040842

DEDICATION

This book, *100 Ways to Kill Cancer* is dedicated to help cancer patients better understand the fundamental causes of human malignancies and how breakthroughs in laboratory and clinical researches have achieve several new life-saving treatments. We hope this book can help readers overcome the fear towards malignancies, knowing that new progresses are accomplished almost daily by dedicated researchers and physicians. Even better, we want to inspire new generation of future scientists to invent their own new ways in treating cancer for ultimate eradication of the disease.

CONTENTS

ACKNOWLEDGMENTS

CHAPTER I: Destroy the DNA

1. Introduction
2. The Brick-and-Mortar of DNA Replication
3. Killing Cancer Cells by Strangling Their DNA strands
4. Destroyed the microtubule, no winner in the tug-of-war
5. Alkylating agents, bumpy road for DNA replication
6. Histone acetylation, revive tumor suppressors
7. PARP inhibitors – the key to keeping broken DNA strands apart

CHAPTER II: Shut Off the Pipeline

1. Introduction
2. The "Warburg effect", from imaging to therapeutic targeting
3. Angiogenesis inhibitors, cutting off cancers' supply lines
4. Chicken or the Egg: IDH mutations and Tumorigenesis
5. Depriving cancer of essential amino acids
6. Shutting down the recycling center via proteasome inhibition

CHAPTER III: Push for Differentiation

1. Introduction
2. Pushing cancer cells back to its differentiated status
3. Eradicating cancer stem cells, how to get there

Shuhua (Steve) Zheng, Ph.D.

CHAPTER IV: Targeted Therapy

1. Introduction
2. Imatinib (Gleevec) - A paradigm shift in cancer therapy
3. Epidermal growth factor receptor (EGFR) inhibitors - blocking signals by removing the antenna
4. Targeting MAPK pathway: too many mutations, not enough inhibitors
5. Mutations in PI3K pathway, how can we target you?
6. Bcl-2 inhibition, tipping the balance towards cell death

CHAPTER V: Immunotherapy

1. Introduction
2. Adoptive T-cell therapy – Reviving tumor infiltrating T-lymphocytes (TILs)
3. Finding a needle in a haystack – T-cell receptor-engineered T-cell therapy
4. CAR T-cell therapy, a promise for cancer cure?
5. Checkpoint inhibition, making immunotherapy 'off-the-shelf'
6. Cancer vaccine, a light from future for cancer prevention
   DNA

ACKNOWLEDGMENTS

I would like to thank my parents and my sister for their love and continuous support. I would like to thank my fiancé Dr. Yue (Katherine) Meng for her love and support. My appreciation also goes to the editor of this book Mr. James Hong. I would extend my appreciation for my Ph.D. training in the Cancer Biology program in University of Miami, Miller School of Medicine, under the meticulous guidance of Dr. Julio C. Barredo. I am currently enrolled as a medical student in Nova Southeastern University, College of Medicine (NSU-COM). I thank NSU-COM for the ongoing medical training and education.

Most importantly, the content in this book is a brief introduction of scientific achievements in cancer research. I would like to thank researchers and physicians for their relentless effort in finding better cures for human malignancies. We are trying our best to include as many citations for a specific topic as possible. However, due to limited space, some groundbreaking publications on a specific topic may not be cited in this book.

CHAPTER I: DESTROY THE DNA

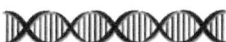

"Towards the end of his life, the German biologist Theodor Boveri (1862–1915) published a prophetic and much-quoted manuscript on the genetic basis of cancer."

Christopher J. Lord, Ph.D.

"... that cancer and diseases of aging are two sides of the DNA-damage problem."

Jan H.J. Hoeijmakers, Ph.D.

"In light of the recent data strongly hinting that much of late-stage cancer's untreatability may arise from its possession of too many antioxidants..."

James Watson, Ph.D.

Shuhua (Steve) Zheng, Ph.D.

Introduction

In 1910s, the German biologist Theodor Boveri first proposed that alterations in the chromosome constitution might be the driving factor for tumorigenesis, a hypothesis that became well proven one century after his death. Changes in the structure and constitution of chromosomes take place during embryonic development that allows a single stem cell to become a whole human body. The chromosome modification process possibly occurs by turning 'on' and 'off' gene expression so that cells can adapt to different living conditions and differentiation stages. This process is strictly regulated and cells that fail to follow these regulatory rules are often guided toward apoptosis (a highly organized, non-inflammatory way of cell death).

Genetic instability refers to the increased rate of genetic alterations throughout a cell's life cycle. This process, for example, can turn on the expression of embryonic genes in well-differentiated (cells that have fully committed to a specific type) tissue cells that leads to the generation of poorly differentiated cancer-like cells. These genes are often grouped into several types based on their function. Oncogenes are a group of genes that upregulated expression can cause transformation of healthy tissue to malignant cells via uncontrolled cell proliferation. In healthy tissue cells, the expression of oncogenes are suppressed via tumor suppressor genes to make sure cell proliferation and division are fine-tuned and under control. Genetic instability can lead to direct upregulation of oncogene expression or it may create new genes via ligation of DNA fragments. At the same time, the expression of tumor suppressors can be destroyed or shut down. All these changes may eventually lead to malignant cells with unlimited capacity of proliferation if they do not undergo apoptosis.

Ironically, one major strategy to kill cancer cells is to essentially destruct their genomes. The idea is that with significant accumulation of genetic defects in cancer cells, their DNA repair machinery will become overwhelmed and cause apoptosis. However, for malignant cells that avoided apoptosis despite their genetic instability, will chemotherapy be capable of inducing further genetic destruction to cause cell death? While most chemotherapeutic agents can cause significant DNA damage in cancer cells, they usually come with deleterious side effects since healthy tissue cells also rely on their DNA for survival. Thus, strategies that selectively predispose only cancer cells to genetic damage are critical in improving the therapeutic efficacy of chemotherapeutic agents and radiation therapy as well. Fortunately, scientists have brought new hope to solve this conundrum with the development of compounds such as PARP inhibitors that function by diminishing the genetic repair capability of cancer cells to make them vulnerable to chemotherapy.

The million-dollar question is why does our body's immune system fail to remove cancer cells on its own? Normal cells that accumulate genetic damage either undergo apoptosis or are removed by our immune system. Researches have shown that execution of either of these mechanisms is mainly dependent on the generation of reactive oxygen species (ROS) including superoxide, hydrogen peroxide, hydroxyl ions, etc. Indeed, some DNA-damaging agents used therapeutically also require ROS to trigger apoptosis. If we consume a surplus of antioxidants in our diet, it may promote the survival of cells with genetic alterations or help develop

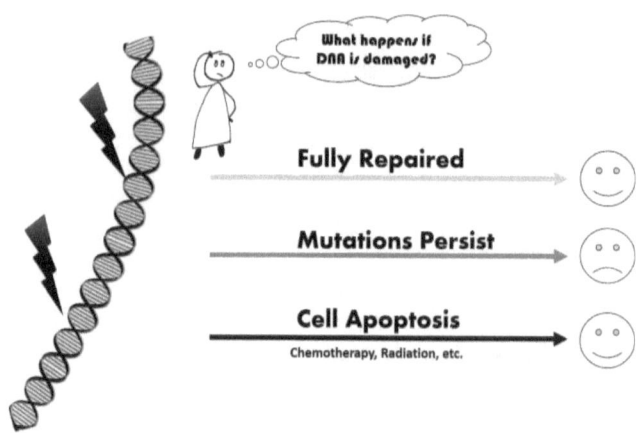

Figure 1.1: DNA damages can occur spontaneously or be induced by treatments for cancer. Damages that are fully repaired will not cause genetic mutations, whereas unrepaired damages can lead to malignancies. Massive DNA damages induced by some cancer treatments will usually cause cell death.

resistance against anti-cancer therapies. Concerned with the potential involvement of antioxidants in tumorigenesis, Dr. Watson, the Nobel Prize winner for the discovery of DNA double helix structure, openly criticizes media promoting the heavy consumption of antioxidants through dietary supplements.

In CHAPTER 1, we will take you on a journey of how cancer cells can be eradicated through various strategies that trigger DNA damage to give readers a taste of these talented ideas.

Reference

1. Lengauer C, Kinzler KW, Vogelstein B. Genetic instabilities in human cancers. Nature. 1998 Dec 17;396(6712):643-9.
2. Watson J. Oxidants, antioxidants and the current incurability of metastatic cancers. Open Biol. 2013 Jan 8;3(1):120144.
3. Kulms D, Zeise E, Pöppelmann B, Schwarz T. DNA damage, death receptor activation and reactive oxygen species contribute to ultraviolet radiation-induced apoptosis in an essential and independent way. Oncogene. 2002 Aug 29;21(38):5844-51.
4. Chen X, Song M, Zhang B, Zhang Y. Reactive Oxygen Species Regulate T Cell Immune Response in the Tumor Microenvironment. Oxid Med Cell Longev. 2016;2016:1580967.
5. Gelmon KA, Tischkowitz M, Mackay H, Swenerton K, Robidoux A, Tonkin K, Hirte H, Huntsman D, Clemons M, Gilks B, Yerushalmi R, Macpherson E, Carmichael J, Oza A. Olaparib in patients with recurrent high-grade serous or poorly differentiated ovarian carcinoma or triple-negative breast cancer: a phase 2, multicentre, open-label, non-randomised study. Lancet Oncol. 2011 Sep;12(9):852-61.

Shuhua (Steve) Zheng, Ph.D.

The Brick-and-Mortar of DNA Replication

Cancer cells tend to divide faster than their normal healthy counterparts. To fuel their rapid rate of cell division, cancer cells are in constant need of DNA building blocks called nucleotides. There are four types of nucleotides – Adenine (A), Thymine (T), Guanine (G), and Cytosine (C). Tumor cells are in constant need of those building bricks to make copies of its genome whereas most normal tissues cells don't need as much since they are slow cycling cells.

Based on this principle, scientists developed a class of drugs called nucleotide analogs. These analogs are similar enough in structure to A, T, G or C that malignant cells incorporate them, but ultimately interrupt DNA replication altogether upon doing so. Halting DNA replication triggers programmed cell death scientifically known as apoptosis. This strategy is similar to entering a broken code into a computer program. Running said program will cause the program to collapse. Albeit being developed decades ago, nucleotide analogs show continued success in treating cancer and new drugs that are being developed are still based on the original mechanism.

One of the most popular nucleotide analogs for cancer treatment is the cytosine analog, Cytarabine (Ara-C), which is commonly used to treat acute myelogenous and lymphoblastic leukemias. Cancer cells metabolize Ara-C into its active form, which becomes incorporated during DNA replication. Activated Ara-C terminates further nucleotide addition, thus inhibits DNA replication and triggers apoptosis in cancer cells. The partially synthesized DNA fragments will trigger a potentially toxic progress called DNA damage response which will eventually kill the malignant cells. Other nucleotide analogs commonly used include Fludarabine, Cladribine, Gemcitabine, Fluorouracil, Clofarabine and Capecitabine that work similarly to Cytarabine that cancer cells will mistakenly incorporate into its DNA during replication.

Because most normal tissue cells do not have as high of a demand for building blocks, they are not as significantly affected by nucleotide analogs. However, this strategy is far from perfection because there are tissue cells that undergo constant turnover such as skin cells, cells in blood circulation, and intestinal lining cells. Because of their high regeneration rate, these cells are susceptible to the effects of the nucleotide analogs. As a result, cancer patients who are treated with this class of anti-cancer drugs inevitably experience some unfavorable side effects in these areas of body. To bypass this obstacle, multiple clinical trials are taking place to test a combinational treatment of various therapeutic agents with nucleotide analogs that will hopefully improve the therapeutic efficiency and offset the side effects of standalone nucleotide analogs.

Another class of anti-tumor drugs is antimetabolites, which use a different method to inhibit cell division in cancer cells by inhibiting the synthesis of nucleotide building blocks. Anti-tumor drugs that works based on this strategy are generally grouped as antimetabolites. Methotrexate is an antimetabolite that has been used to treat cancer since the 1950s and is still one of the most popular anti-tumor drugs prescribed today. Its mechanism involves inhibiting a key enzyme called dihydrofolate reductase (DHFR), which is required to generate nucleotide Thymidine (T). However, cancer cells can evade this inhibitory effect by shutting down

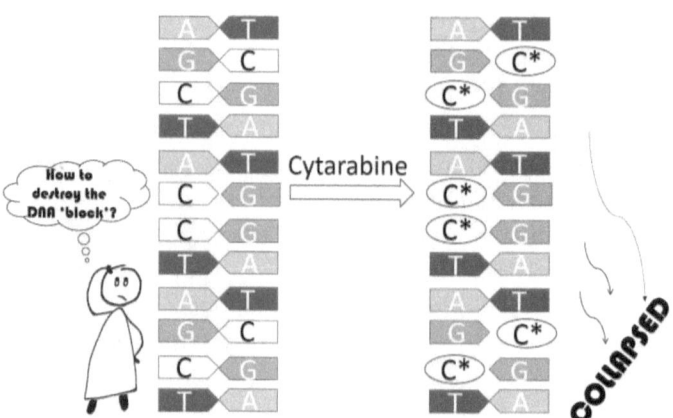

Figure 1.2: Cytarabine, a type of nucleotide analog, can be mistakenly incorporated into the DNA of cancer cells during DNA replication. This process will alter the structure of DNA helix, causing significant amount of DNA damages and eventually lead to cancer cell death.

methotrexate transporters in the cell membrane, promoting efflux (export) of methotrexate, or by increasing its expression of DHFR. A more recently developed drug called Pemetrexed simultaneously inhibits more than 3 enzymes involved in the generation of nucleotides. Because multiple enzymes are inhibited simultaneously, cancer cells are less likely to develop resistance mechanisms to Pemetrexed as compared with Methotrexate.

To recap, if we compare cell division to construction and nucleotides to rectangular bricks we know and normally use, nucleotide analogs can be thought as bricks with defects. If used, analogs will compromise the structural integrity during the construction process and will lead to utter collapse as we shown in the picture. On the other hand, antimetabolites act as jackhammers destroying the supply of the building blocks, making cancer cells incapable to completing the construction of DNA required for generation of new cancer cells.

Reference

1. Galmarini CM, Mackey JR, Dumontet C. Nucleoside analogues and nucleobases in cancer treatment. Lancet Oncol. 2002 Jul;3(7):415-24.
2. Jordheim LP, Durantel D, Zoulim F, Dumontet C. Advances in the development of nucleoside and nucleotide analogues for cancer and viral diseases. Nat Rev Drug Discov. 2013 Jun;12(6):447-64. doi: 10.1038/nrd4010.
3. Cai J, Damaraju VL, Groulx N, Mowles D, Peng Y, Robins MJ, Cass CE, Gros P. Two distinct molecular mechanisms underlying cytarabine resistance in human leukemic cells. Cancer Res. 2008 Apr 1;68(7):2349-57. doi: 10.1158/0008-5472.CAN-07-5528.
4. Candoni A, Papayannidis C, Martinelli G, Simeone E, Gottardi M, Iacobucci I, Gherlinzoni F, Visani G, Baccarani M, Fanin R. Flai (fludarabine, cytarabine, idarubicin) plus low-dose gemtuzumab ozogamicin as induction therapy in cd33-positive aml: Final results and long term outcome of a phase ii multicenter clinical trial. Am J Hematol. 2018 Feb 2. doi: 10.1002/ajh.25057
5. Löwenberg B, Pabst T, Vellenga E, van Putten W, Schouten HC, Graux C, Ferrant A, Sonneveld P, Biemond BJ, Gratwohl A, de Greef GE, Verdonck LF, Schaafsma MR, Gregor M, Theobald M, Schanz U, Maertens J, Ossenkoppele GJ; Dutch-Belgian Cooperative Trial Group for Hemato-Oncology (HOVON) and Swiss Group for Clinical Cancer Research (SAKK) Collaborative Group. Cytarabine dose for acute myeloid leukemia. N Engl J Med. 2011 Mar 17;364(11):1027-36. doi: 10.1056/NEJMoa1010222.

6. Adjei AA. Pharmacology and mechanism of action of pemetrexed. Clin Lung Cancer. 2004 Apr;5 Suppl 2:S51-5.
7. Kaye SB. New antimetabolites in cancer chemotherapy and their clinical impact. Br J Cancer. 1998;78 Suppl 3:1-7.
8. Hagner N, Joerger M. Cancer chemotherapy: targeting folic acid synthesis. Cancer Manag Res. 2010 Nov 19;2:293-301. doi: 10.2147/CMR.S10043.

Killing Cancer Cells by Strangling Their DNA strands

DNA consists of two complementary strands that wind together in the form of a spiral staircase. Each step of the staircase represents a binding between complement nucleotides on each strand. DNA replication is a complicated energy-exhaustive process that involves various enzymes. These enzymes "walk" across nucleotide by nucleotide to ensure the newly formed copy has the exact same genetic information as the original template. Duplex DNA is further organized into loops that consist of areas that are either more twisted (positive supercoil) or less twisted (negative supercoil).

During replication, the DNA duplex is constantly unwound to expose its nucleotides to the replication enzymes. Unwinding DNA causes the un-replicated portion to become more twisted. The positive supercoil eventually makes further unwinding impossible thus halting DNA replication. To prevent this from happening, a group of enzymes called topoisomerases cut the DNA in the un-replicated regions to release the torsion generated by the over-twisted DNA strands.

The same process of DNA unwinding is also used during DNA transcription for protein synthesis. Due to the higher rate of DNA replication in cancer cells, this process can be targeted therapeutically for cancer treatments. Such treatments involve disrupting topoisomerases, which halts DNA replication, causing its strands to become supercoiled with accumulation of incomplete RNA transcripts. As you can imagine, an accumulation of such events induces a potent toxic response that eventually leads to cancer cell death.

Topoisomerase inhibitors such as daunorubicin and doxorubicin have been used as potent antitumor drugs since the 1950s. They were first discovered in bacteria and are now used as first line drug therapy in treating multiple types of cancer which include, but are not limited to acute leukemia, breast cancer, and Hodgkin's lymphomas.

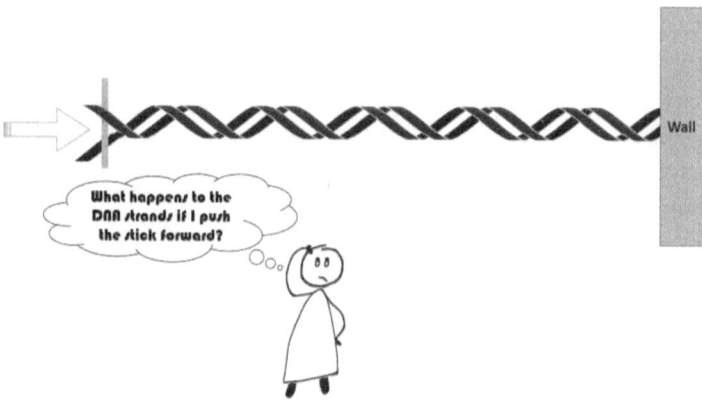

Figure 1.3: DNA strands can be 'unwinded' by toposisomerases during replication. This process is inhibited by topoisomerase inhibitors, generating 'strangled' DNAs that can trigger cell death.

However, one major side effect from the use of topoisomerase inhibitor drugs is cardiotoxicity. Patients who are treated with a high dosage for a long period of time can experience heart failure. Scientists discovered that metabolizing these drugs in our bodies generate free radicals (hydrogen peroxide and hydroxyl radical) in the muscle cells of the heart. Heart muscle cells heavily depend on the oxidative metabolism to generate energy needed to pump the heart. This makes them vulnerable to the accumulation of free oxidative radicals formed from the metabolism of doxorubicin/daunorubicin.

Can antioxidants reduce the side effects of topoisomerase inhibitor drugs? Several studies have preclinical data showing antioxidant compounds (e.g. probucol, flavonoid, carvedilol, etc.) can protect heart muscle cells from the damage of doxorubicin/daunorubicin-induced oxidative stress, whereas the antioxidant vitamin E is generally ineffective. Potential novel strategies that use renin-angiotensin system blockade, beta-blockers, and iron chelator Dexrazoxane are also undergoing preclinical studies. Given the large amount of cancer patients treated with doxorubicin/daunorubicin, antioxidants may reduce the chance of developing cardiac problems. Meanwhile, isomers (structurally and functionally similar compounds) of these first-generation topoisomerases inhibitors are constantly under development and clinical trials that will hopefully generate similar antitumor efficacy with much lower toxicity.

Reference:
1. Cardinale D, Colombo A, Bacchiani G, Tedeschi I, Meroni CA, Veglia F, Civelli M, Lamantia G, Colombo N, Curigliano G, Fiorentini C, Cipolla CM. Early detection of anthracycline cardiotoxicity and improvement with heart failure therapy. Circulation. 2015 Jun 2;131(22):1981-8.
2. Kaiserová H, Simůnek T, van der Vijgh WJ, Bast A, Kvasnicková E. Flavonoids as protectors against doxorubicin cardiotoxicity: role of iron chelation, antioxidant activity and inhibition of carbonyl reductase. Biochim Biophys Acta. 2007 Sep;1772(9):1065-74.

3. Singal PK, Siveski-Iliskovic N, Hill M, Thomas TP, Li T. Combination therapy with probucol prevents adriamycin-induced cardiomyopathy. J Mol Cell Cardiol. 1995 Apr;27(4):1055-63.
4. Panchuk R, Skorokhyd N, Chumak V, Lehka L, Omelyanchik S, Gurinovich V, Moiseenok A, Heffeter P, Berger W, Stoika R. Specific antioxidant compounds differentially modulate cytotoxic activity of doxorubicin and cisplatin: in vitro and in vivo study. Croat Med J. 2014 Jun 1;55(3):206-17.
5. Chatterjee K, Zhang J, Honbo N, Karliner JS. Doxorubicin cardiomyopathy. Cardiology. 2010;115(2):155-62.
6. Volkova M, Russell R 3rd. Anthracycline cardiotoxicity: prevalence, pathogenesis and treatment. Curr Cardiol Rev. 2011 Nov;7(4):214-20.

Destroyed the microtubule, no winner in the tug-of-war

In order for malignant cells to multiply, they must first replicate their DNA to secure a copy of its original DNA for its new cells. DNA replication requires the use of tube-like structures, called microtubules, to pull apart the newly synthesized DNA so that the resulting two daughter cells have an equal amount of chromatin respectively. Microtubules themselves consist of individual tubulin units that are made of protein and congregate to form a spindle-like structure to perform its intended function.

After the chromatin become separated, the spindle disintegrates, and the microtubules (return) to either their monomer form or become a part of the cytoskeleton, which maintains the shape and integrity of cells. Because malignant cells replicate rapidly, the process of assembling and disassembling of the microtubule spindle occurs at a much faster rate than that of most normal tissue cells. This makes cancer cells vulnerable to drugs that either inhibit the formation or destabilize the microtubule spindle, which prevent the production of a functional spindle, thus inhibiting cell proliferation. Based on this principle, various chemotherapeutic agents have been developed.

One class of such drugs destabilize the microtubule spindle is the Vinca alkaloids (e.g. Vincristine), which are synthesized from the Madagascar periwinkle plant. This group of drugs kill cancer cells by interacting with the tubulin units to stop them from polymerizing. Another drug class functions by stabilizing microtubules, which shuts down tubulin turnover and renders cancer cells unable to form new spindles. This group of drugs is best represented by paclitaxel (Taxol®), synthesized from a compound found in the Taxus wallichiana plant that was approved by the FDA in 1992. However, due to its widespread use for cancer treatment and research, the Taxus wallichiana has been listed as an endangered species since 2011. To work around this, derivatives of paclitaxel are currently being developed and under clinical trials.

One major clinical conundrum associated with use of microtubule inhibitor drugs is that cancer cells may develop resistance to the aforementioned drugs. For instance, tumor cells treated with paclitaxel can switch to

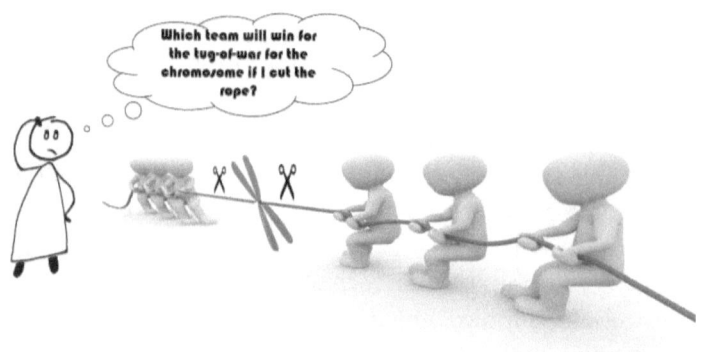

Figure 1.4: Proper separation of chromatids after DNA replication is required for cancer cell proliferation. Microtubules attached to centromeres of chromatids will help make sure each daughter cells will have a complete set of chromosomes. Drugs that either inhibit microtubule formation or promote its disassemble will thus inhibit cancer cell proliferation.

a different type of tubulin that paclitaxel cannot stably bind to. Cancer cells can also mutate their tubulin units to generate less stable microtubules to form paclitaxel-resistant tumor cells. Resistance to Vincristine has also been reported via the activation of Multidrug Resistance-Associated Protein 1 (MRP1) in cancer cells that results in increasing the export of the drug thus mitigating its effects.

To combat this, new classes of microtubule inhibitors that thwart drug resistance are currently under development. Epothilones, a microtubule stabilizer drug class, were shown to be capable of overcoming paclitaxel resistance related to tubulin mutations. Vinflunines, a new microtubule destabilizer drug, are shown better absorbed to increase the intracellular concentration to generate more potent antitumor effects.

Reference:
1. Moudi M, Go R, Yien CY, Nazre M. Vinca alkaloids. Int J Prev Med. 2013 Nov;4(11):1231-5.
2. Cao YN, Zheng LL, Wang D, Liang XX, Gao F, Zhou XL. Recent advances in microtubule-stabilizing agents. Eur J Med Chem. 2018 Jan 1;143:806-828. doi: 10.1016/j.ejmech.2017.11.062.
3. Thomas, P. & Farjon, A. 2011. Taxus wallichiana. The IUCN Red List of Threatened Species 2011: e.T46171879A9730085. http://dx.doi.org/10.2305/IUCN.UK.2011-2.RLTS.T46171879A9730085.en.
4. Perez EA. Microtubule inhibitors: Differentiating tubulin-inhibiting agents based on mechanisms of action, clinical activity, and resistance. Mol Cancer Ther. 2009 Aug;8(8):2086-95. doi: 10.1158/1535-7163.MCT-09-0366.
5. Orr GA, Verdier-Pinard P, McDaid H, Horwitz SB. Mechanisms of Taxol resistance related to microtubules.

Oncogene. 2003 Oct 20;22(47):7280-95.
6. Gonçalves A, Braguer D, Kamath K, Martello L, Briand C, Horwitz S, Wilson L, Jordan MA. Resistance to Taxol in lung cancer cells associated with increased microtubule dynamics. Proc Natl Acad Sci U S A. 2001 Sep 25;98(20):11737-42.

Alkylating agents, bumpy road for DNA replication

Alkylating agents are one of the oldest classes of chemotherapeutic drugs that are still on the frontline battle against multiple types of cancers. The anti-tumor activities of this group of compounds were first systematically investigated during World War II when studies revealed naval personnel exposed to mustard gas experienced therapeutic effects against cancer. Scientists later discovered that the nitrogen mustards in mustard gas attributed to the anti-tumor effects seen in soldiers due to its DNA alkylating activities.

Instead of 'tricking' cancer cells incorporating nucleotide analog when the cells are conducting DNA replication and transcription, alkylating agents directly modify the genome of cancer cells by adding alkyl groups (C_nH_{2n+1}) to the nucleotides in their DNA strands. This process leads to several changes in the properties of the nucleotides. For example, the modified nucleotide may no longer be able to base-pair with its partner during DNA synthesis, causing a mismatch in the DNA double-helix. The added alkyl groups also "stick out" from the normally "smooth" DNA helix, which halts the sliding of enzymes involved in DNA replication and transcription along the DNA helix. These disruptions in DNA replication and transcription in alkylated DNA strand subsequently lead to generation of broken DNA strands, triggering apoptosis. DNA alkylation is similar to occurrence of obstacles and potholes during driving (sliding of enzymes), making the driving experience uncomfortable and can eventually stop the vehicle if the destructions are significant enough. Alkylating agents can also crosslink different strands of DNA, making it difficult for repair enzymes to fix the broken DNA strands. This causes the "road trip" to be more adventurous for the enzymes involved in DNA replication and transcription.

Popular alkylating drugs used in cancer treatment include cisplatin, carmustine, cyclophosphamide, mitomycin C, and the more recently FDA-approved temozolomide. However popular, DNA alkylation can also occur in healthy cells and cause DNA damage. This leads to unwanted side effects such as hematopoietic toxicity, gastrointestinal toxicity, and higher chances of acquiring secondary tumors due to treatment-related accumulation of genetic mutations.

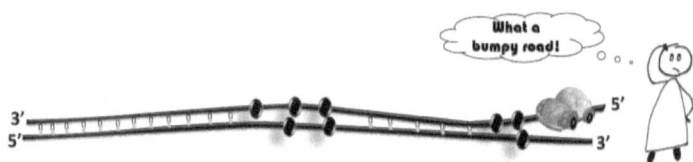

Figure 1.5: The nucleotides in the DNA can be alkylated directly by treatment of alkylating agents. Alkylation will alter the structure of nucleotides and thus will impair the base pairing between nucleotides.

Scientists have developed several strategies to modify alkylating agents to be more selective against cancer cells to offset the aforementioned side-effects. For example, the original cisplatin design was improved by wrapping it with lipids to generate nanoparticles called liposomal cisplatin (Lipoplatin). Lipoplatin is more penetrable in the leaky vasculatures of solid tumors and clinical studies have shown up to 200-fold higher accumulation of Lipoplatin in solid tumors as compared with adjacent normal tissue, demonstrating increased selectivity. Thus, the general toxicity associated with original cisplatin has been significantly reduced. Other preclinical trials are studying embedded antibodies that can specifically recognize cancer cells to selectively deliver vesicles that carry cisplatin. With all these advancements, we will see more tumor-specific alkylating agents in an oncologist's toolkit in the near future.

Reference

1. Adair FE, Bagg HJ. EXPERIMENTAL AND CLINICAL STUDIES ON THE TREATMENT OF CANCER BY DICHLORETHYLSULPHIDE (MUSTARD GAS. Ann Surg. 1931 Jan;93(1):190-9.
2. Chaney SG, Sancar A. DNA repair: enzymatic mechanisms and relevance to drug response. J Natl Cancer Inst. 1996 Oct 2;88(19):1346-60.
3. Deans AJ, West SC. DNA interstrand crosslink repair and cancer. Nat Rev Cancer. 2011 Jun 24;11(7):467-80.
4. Zhu P, Du XL, Lu G, Zhu JJ. Survival benefit of glioblastoma patients after FDA approval of temozolomide concomitant with radiation and bevacizumab: A population-based study. Oncotarget. 2017 Jul 4;8(27):44015-44031
5. Deshpande PP, Biswas S, Torchilin VP. Current trends in the use of liposomes for tumor targeting. Nanomedicine (Lond). 2013 Sep;8(9):1509-28.
6. Hawkins MM, Wilson LM, Burton HS, Potok MH, Winter DL, Marsden HB, Stovall MA. Radiotherapy, Alkylating Agents, and Risk of Bone Cancer After Childhood Cancer. J Natl Cancer Inst. 1996 Mar 6;88(5):270-8.
7. Dhar S, Gu FX, Langer R, Farokhzad OC, Lippard SJ. Targeted delivery of cisplatin to prostate cancer cells by aptamer functionalized Pt(IV) prodrug-PLGA-PEG nanoparticles. Proc Natl Acad Sci U S A. 2008 Nov 11;105(45):17356-61

Shuhua (Steve) Zheng, Ph.D.

Histone acetylation, revive tumor suppressors

While alkylating agents make DNA strands bulky and prone to damage, there is another group of compounds that can modify DNA strands in such a way that tumor suppressor genes can be re-exposed for transcription. The promoter region of tumor suppressors genes is often made inaccessible during tumorigenesis via a process called histone de-acetylation. This deacetylated region in the DNA is often further modified by another process called methylation. These coupled processes hide certain regions of DNA from the binding of transcription factors, leading to the silencing of tumor suppressors. Based on our understanding of how tumor suppressors are downregulated in malignant cells, two strategies were developed to release the inhibition and revive the transcription of tumor suppressor.

The first strategy to revive tumor suppressors is to directly inhibit the enzymes responsible for histone deacetylation, i.e., histone deacetylases (HDACs). The inhibitors that specifically target HDACs are called HDAC inhibitor (HDACi) including vorinostat, romidepsin and the more recently approved panobinostat and belinostat. HDACi treatment release the structural hindrance in the promoter region of tumor suppressors so that transcriptional factors can bind and upregulate gene expression. Meanwhile, for unknown reasons, the expression of oncogenes are also concurrently downregulated with HDACi treatment. Consequently, HDAC treatment significantly increases the amount of tumor suppressors available, thus overwhelming cancer cells eventually leading to their death.

In addition to the proteins directly involved in cell

survival, HDACi treatment also promotes terminal differentiation of cancer cells via reactivation of differentiation factors. As we will discuss later, suppression of proteins that mediate terminal differentiation can also help cancer cells escape contact inhibition that allows them to proliferate. With HDACi

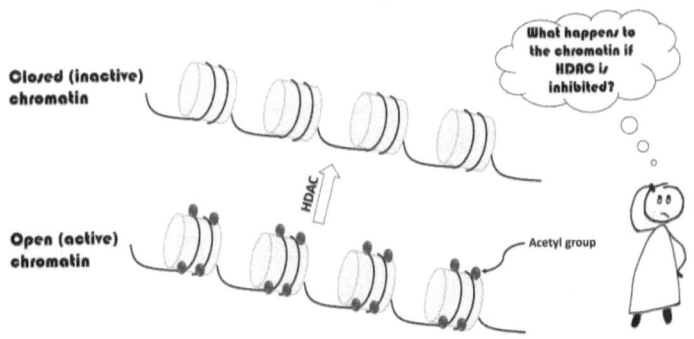

Figure 1.6: Acetylation of histones will help the DNA strands accessible to transcription factors. On the other hand, methylation of histones will impede the binding of transcription factors. Inhibition of histone deacetylases (HDACs) will make DNA sequence adopt an 'open structure' and thus facilitating the transcription of tumor suppressor genes.

treatment, the transcription of proteins that mediate cell differentiation are reactivated, which inhibits cancer cell proliferation and curb cancer growth.

As discussed, deacetylation of histones in the promoter region of tumor suppressors lead to increased methylation. Histones are responsible for packaging the DNA into a condensed form that occludes access from transcription factors. Consequently, another strategy that reverses this process is via direct inhibition of DNA methyltransferases (DNMTs), enzymes that mediate histone methylation. DNMT inhibitors, including azacytidine and decitabine, also reactivate the expression of tumor suppressors and cause tumor cell death. It is important to note here that the anti-tumor effects of both azacytidine and decitabine are attributed by the fact that they are nucleotide analogs. Their anti-DNMT mechanisms are still under investigation.

Now, from what we know about the therapeutic mechanisms of HDAC and DNMT inhibitors, the combined treatment of these drugs has even stronger effects in reviving the expression of tumor suppressors. DNMT inhibitors promote demethylation of histones, which then get acetylated/activated by the presence of HDACi, ultimately reviving the expression of tumor suppressors. This process is similar to resurfacing roads. First, DNMT inhibitors remove the old surface (demethylation) and HDACi puts on a new surface (acetylation). This leads to a more efficient movement of traffic (upregulation of tumor suppressor transcription). Indeed, the efficacy of this strategy in treating cancer is substantiated by preclinical studies and multiple clinical trials that are in place that combine HDAC and DNMT inhibitors.

Reference

1. Stresemann C, Lyko F. Modes of action of the DNA methyltransferase inhibitors azacytidine and decitabine. Int J Cancer. 2008 Jul 1;123(1):8-13.
2. Ahuja N, Sharma AR, Baylin SB. Epigenetic Therapeutics: A New Weapon in the War Against Cancer. Annu Rev Med. 2016;67:73-89.
3. Ghoshal K, Datta J, Majumder S, Bai S, Dong X, Parthun M, Jacob ST. Inhibitors of histone deacetylase and DNA methyltransferase synergistically activate the methylated metallothionein I promoter by activating the transcription factor MTF-1 and forming an open chromatin structure. Mol Cell Biol. 2002 Dec;22(23):8302-19.
4. Peart MJ, Smyth GK, van Laar RK, Bowtell DD, Richon VM, Marks PA, Holloway AJ, Johnstone RW. Identification and functional significance of genes regulated by structurally different histone deacetylase inhibitors. Proc Natl Acad Sci U S A. 2005 Mar 8;102(10):3697-702.
5. Pathania R, Ramachandran S, Mariappan G, Thakur P, Shi H, Choi JH, Manicassamy S, Kolhe R, Prasad PD, Sharma S, Lokeshwar BL, Ganapathy V, Thangaraju M. Combined Inhibition of DNMT and HDAC Blocks the Tumorigenicity of Cancer Stem-like Cells and Attenuates Mammary Tumor Growth. Cancer Res. 2016 Jun 1;76(11):3224-35.
6. Morera L, Lübbert M, Jung M. Targeting histone methyltransferases and demethylases in clinical trials for cancer therapy. Clin Epigenetics. 2016 May 24;8:57.

Shuhua (Steve) Zheng, Ph.D.

PARP inhibitors – the key to keeping broken DNA strands apart

Because the exposed ends of broken DNA are toxic to mammalian cells, evolution has developed a very delicate and efficient mechanism of locating the damage and recruiting proteins that selectively repair said DNA damage. This mechanism is constantly active to keep our genome intact to prevent the accumulation of DNA damage that occurs during social activities such as sunbathing or drinking alcohol. Cells that are able to withstand such heavy unrepaired DNA damage mutate into malignant 'immortal' cells that we know today as cancer cells. As efficient as this DNA damage repair mechanism is, if a significant amount of DNA damage occurs within a short period of time, it can overwhelm the DNA damage repair system, leading to the triggering of apoptosis and cell death.

The idea behind current cancer treatments is to overwhelm the DNA repair machinery using strategies previously discussed such as microtubule inhibitors, topoisomerase inhibitors, or nucleotide analogs to kill the malignant cells. Consequently, the inhibition of the DNA damage repair system leaves broken DNA strands unrepaired, thus triggering cancer cell death. The first step in repairing damaged DNA is to detect where the damage is located within the genome, a process mainly mediated by a protein called poly ADP ribose polymerase (PARP). PARP usually binds to single-stranded broken DNA and consequently signals the recruitment of DNA repair enzymes to fix the damage. PARP's main role is to initiate DNA repair, making it a desirable target for chemotherapy. However, it is only recently that the FDA

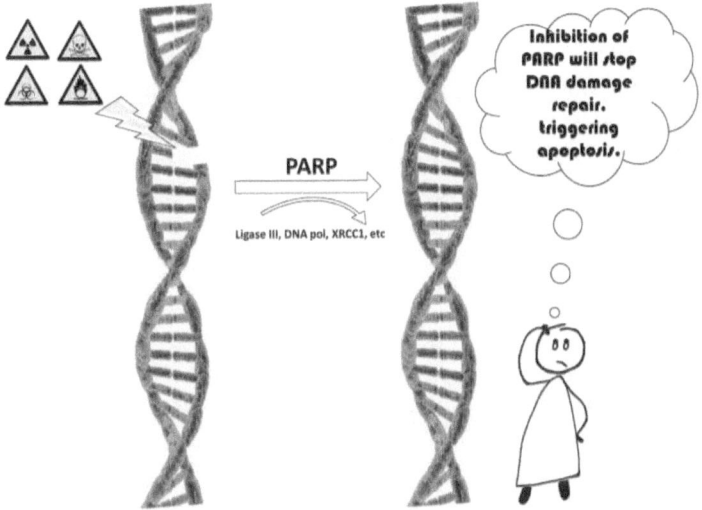

Figure 1.7: PARP is involved in repair of damaged DNA. By doing so, PARP inhibitors will potentiate the efficacy of therapeutic agents (chemotherapy, radiotherapy) that trigger cancer death by inducing DNA damage.

approved the use of PARP inhibitors, such as rucaparib, for advanced ovarian cancer, and olaparib, for metastatic breast cancer in 2016 and 2018, respectively.

This is not to say that the idea of combining PARP inhibitors with DNA damage-inducing agents to efficiently kill cancer cell was only recently thought of. In fact, the majority of successful clinical trials were initially conducted using the combination of PARP inhibitors with DNA damage-inducing agents like paclitaxel, cisplatin and carboplatin. These trials have shown the addition of PARP inhibitors potentiated the cytotoxic effects of paclitaxel/cisplatin/carboplatin-induced DNA damage, leading to more efficient apoptosis induction.

It is worth noting that although current radiation therapy mainly functions by inducing DNA damage, it is conceivable that the addition of PARP inhibitors may also potentiate the efficacy of radiotherapy as well. The efficacy of PARP as a radiosensitizer has been proven in multiple preclinical studies, although the extent of side effects that occur due to this treatment strategy in real patients have yet to be studied.

Reference

1. Javle M, Curtin NJ. The role of PARP in DNA repair and its therapeutic exploitation. Br J Cancer. 2011 Oct 11;105(8):1114-22.
2. Wilson RH, Evans TJ, Middleton MR, Molife LR, Spicer J, Dieras V, Roxburgh P, Giordano H, Jaw-Tsai S, Goble S, Plummer R. A phase I study of intravenous and oral rucaparib in combination with chemotherapy in patients with advanced solid tumours. Br J Cancer. 2017 Mar 28;116(7):884-892.
3. Oza AM, Cibula D, Benzaquen AO, Poole C, Mathijssen RH, Sonke GS, Colombo N, Špaček J, Vuylsteke P, Hirte H, Mahner S, Plante M, Schmalfeldt B, Mackay H, Rowbottom J, Lowe ES, Dougherty B, Barrett JC, Friedlander M. Olaparib combined with chemotherapy for recurrent platinum-sensitive ovarian cancer: a randomised phase 2 trial. Lancet Oncol. 2015 Jan;16(1):87-97.
4. Sonnenblick A, de Azambuja E, Azim HA Jr, Piccart M. An update on PARP inhibitors--moving to the adjuvant setting. Nat Rev Clin Oncol. 2015 Jan;12(1):27-41.
5. Dizdar O, Arslan C, Altundag K. Advances in PARP inhibitors for the treatment of breast cancer. Expert Opin Pharmacother. 2015;16(18):2751-8.
6. Hastak K, Bhutra S, Parry R, Ford JM. Poly (ADP-ribose) polymerase inhibitor, an effective radiosensitizer in lung and pancreatic cancers. Oncotarget. 2017 Apr 18;8(16):26344-26355.

100 Ways to Kill Cancer

CHAPTER II: SHUT OFF THE PIPELINE

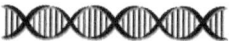

"... what can the causative factors be, and just as often has the idea obtruded itself that the causative factor in the origin of tumors is nothing other than oxygen deficiency"

Otto Heinrich Warburg, M.D., Ph.D.

"Together with glutamine, glucose via glycolysis provides the carbon skeletons, NADPH, and ATP to build new cancer cells..."

Chi Van Dang, M.D., Ph.D.

"If cancer is primarily a disease of energy metabolism, then rational strategies for cancer management should be found in those therapies that specifically target tumor cell energy metabolism."

Thomas N. Seyfried, Ph.D.

Introduction

Given that cancer is a fast-growing mass, you can imagine that cancer cells are constantly competing against healthy cells for nourishment. This takes a toll on our bodies and manifests as initial symptoms such as fatigue and weight loss. Cancer cells fuel their rapid growth via angiogenesis that supplies nutrients required for tumors to increase in size and metastasize. However, these newly generated vessels lack structural integrity, allowing cancer cells to easily perforate the vessel walls and invade other tissues.

Shutting off these "pipelines" can help shrink tumors and potentially curb lethal dissemination of malignant cells. Surgical occlusion of major blood vessels that supply tumor growth is often the treatment of choice to directly remove tumors. Another popular pharmaceutical method to stop tumor growth is to use drugs that specifically inhibit angiogenesis.

High blood glucose levels can also theoretically fuel cancer growth as implicated by studies showing that people with type 2 diabetes have a higher cancer incidence. Because glucose metabolism often generates reactive oxygen species (ROS), a mutagenic group of agents we discussed in Chapter 1, increased glucose uptake could potentially trigger genetic alterations. One would think that because cancer cells are so glucose-hungry, they would metabolize whatever glucose molecule they come across in order to fuel their constant need of energy. In reality, cancer cells barely use glucose for energy production. Instead, most of our absorbed glucose is utilized for the generation of building blocks such as amino acids and nucleotides required for the synthesis of proteins and DNA, respectively. We can compare cancer cells to cars with extremely low MPG due to their inefficient glucose consumption to energy output ratio. This unique trait of cancer cells is called the 'Warburg effect' as we will discuss in more detail in this chapter.

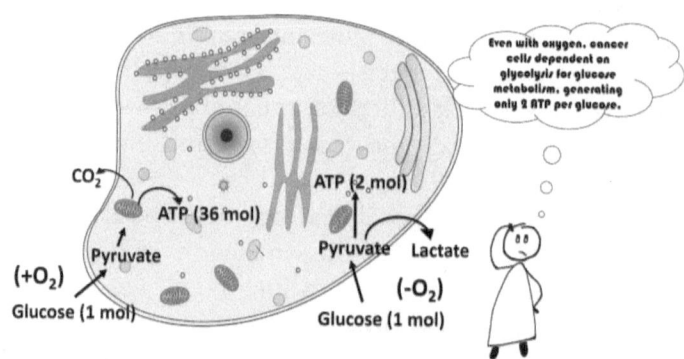

Figure 2.1: Cancer cells are largely dependent on glycolysis for generation of energy (ATP). Compared with TCA cycle that happens in the mitochondria, glycolysis of glucose generate much less APT, making cancer cells vulnerable to disruption of energy supply.

Cars with low fuel efficiency often produce heavy black exhaust due to incomplete combustion of gas that contributes to air pollution. In the case of cancer cells, incomplete metabolism of glucose generates a major 'waste' called lactate, which also "pollutes" surrounding healthy normal tissue. Lactate is an acid end-product of incomplete metabolism that causes our muscles to become sore after strenuous exercise. Massive lactate secretion by cancer cells can acidify the surrounding tissue, leading to several consequences.

The acidic microenvironment caused by tumors can increase their ability to invade healthy tissue, suppress the function of cancer-killing lymphocytes, and cause cancer cells to become resistant to radiation therapy. Some preliminary clinical studies suggest that high serum levels of lactic acid are associated with poor prognosis for certain cancer types. Unfortunately, strategies that involve intervening cancer cells from producing lactate are not been well-established. Some preclinical studies show promise in using bicarbonate (baking soda) to neutralize the acidic tumor microenvironment can, to some degree, curb cancer progression.

Cancer is now being considered a metabolic disease in which both the supply of glucose and its metabolism are critically involved in tumor progression. While scientists have yet to fully understand the potential causal effect of dysregulated glucose metabolism in tumorigenesis, we hope that you will have a better idea of how tumor growth can be therapeutically curbed by intervening its energy supply after reading Chapter 2.

Reference

1. McDonald DM, Baluk P. Significance of blood vessel leakiness in cancer. Cancer Res. 2002 Sep 15;62(18):5381-5.
2. Nishida N, Yano H, Nishida T, Kamura T, Kojiro M. Angiogenesis in cancer. Vasc Health Risk Manag. 2006;2(3):213-9.
3. Giovannucci E, Harlan DM, Archer MC, Bergenstal RM, Gapstur SM, Habel LA, Pollak M, Regensteiner JG, Yee D. Diabetes and cancer: a consensus report. Diabetes Care. 2010 Jul;33(7):1674-85.
4. Dhup S, Dadhich RK, Porporato PE, Sonveaux P. Multiple biological activities of lactic acid in cancer: influences on tumor growth, angiogenesis and metastasis. Curr Pharm Des. 2012;18(10):1319-30.
5. Robey IF, Baggett BK, Kirkpatrick ND, Roe DJ, Dosescu J, Sloane BF, Hashim AI, Morse DL, Raghunand N, Gatenby RA, Gillies RJ. Bicarbonate increases tumor pH and inhibits spontaneous metastases. Cancer Res. 2009 Mar 15;69(6):2260-8.
6. Seyfried TN, Flores RE, Poff AM, D'Agostino DP. Cancer as a metabolic disease: implications for novel therapeutics. Carcinogenesis. 2014 Mar;35(3):515-27.

The "Warburg effect", from imaging to therapeutic targeting

During the 1920s, scientists discovered that cancer cells generate energy differently from their normal counterparts – a phenomenon dubbed the "Warburg effect" after its discover, Dr. Otto Warburg. Before delving deep into biochemical intricacies, the general understanding of the majority of cancer cells is that they require a higher-than-normal amount of glucose to fuel their malignant growth and metastasis. However, scientists have discovered a caveat to their ravenous hunger for glucose.

Cancer cells heavily depend on an inefficient metabolic pathway called glycolysis to generate energy in the form of ATP, the energy currency of all living cells. To dispel any negative connotation with this process, it is important to point out that glycolysis is utilized in almost all healthy living organisms. It is normally used as the first step to break down a molecule of glucose to generate 2 molecules ATP. In a healthy cell, glucose is further broken down in a series of intricate metabolic processes to generate a total of 38 molecules of ATP while producing heat and carbon dioxide. This occurs in what is most infamously known to every high school student in the country as the "powerhouse" of the cell – the mitochondria.

During tumor progression, the normal functions of mitochondria in malignant cells are shut down so that the cells can have more building blocks derived from the intermediates of glucose glycolysis as the main production of building blocks for further growth. As a result, tumor cells demand a higher influx of glucose to meet their energy requirement as opposed to the demands of normal tissue cells.

Based on these discoveries, a tumor-detecting machine called the Positron Emission Tomography (PET) scan was invented in the mid-1970s at the Mallinckrodt Institute of Radiology at Washington University. To detect the presence of tumors, patients first ingest a radioactive glucose analog, 18F-2-fluoro-2-deoxy-D-glucose (FDG), prior to undergoing a PET scan.

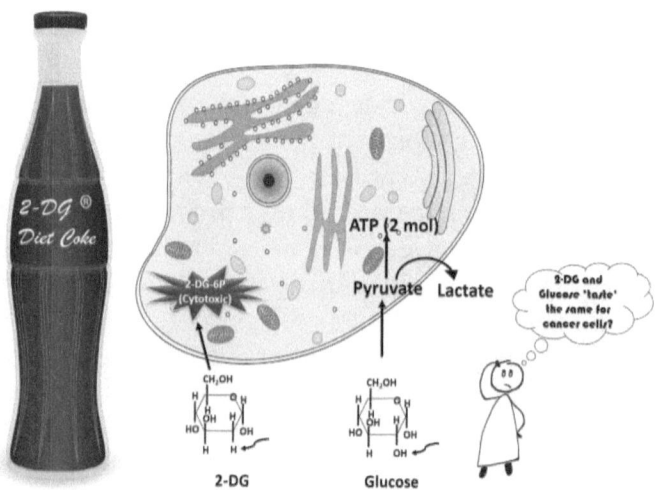

Figure 2.1: Cancer cells have higher demand for energy since they cannot fully metabolize glucose (Warburg effect). Glucose analog s like 2-deoxy-glucose (2-DG) can be taken in by the cancer cells and hijack enzymes required for glucose metabolism.

Malignant cells cannot distinguish between the real glucose or FDG. Since cancer cells requires more energy for survival, more FDG will be taken in as regular molecules of glucose at a much higher rate in cancer cells than normal tissue cells. Using this principle, the PET scan detects the any localizations of FDG signal intensities, which physicians use to determine the location of a tumor and its size. Today, the PET scan is usually supplemented with CT imaging for improved accuracy in differentiating tumor cells from normal tissue cells.

Other types of glucose analogs, including 2-deoxyglucose (2-DG), are instead used as a therapeutic agent. 2-DG is nearly identical in structure to glucose; that cancer cells are tricked to take it in just like normal glucose and try to metabolize through glycolysis. However, after it was phosphorylated by the first enzyme in the glycolysis i.e. hexokinase, the product 2-DG-phosphate cannot be further broken down like its normal counterpart. Thus, when malignant cells ingest 2-DG, it accumulates inside the cells and inhibit further glycolysis, leading to ATP depletion, cell cycle inhibition and ultimately cell death. Recent studies have shown that 2-DG can also disturb protein folding in malignant cells as another means of stopping tumor formation. Because normal tissue cells do not need as much glucose as cancer cells, when treated with glucose analogs like 2-DG, cancer cells will be relatively selected for simultaneous disturbance of energy production and protein folding, leading to their death while leaving normal tissues cells relatively untouched. This strategy is very similar to diet coke or any sugar supplements that tastes sweet and yet has zero calories.

Reference

1. Hamanaka RB, Chandel NS. Targeting glucose metabolism for cancer therapy. J Exp Med. 2012 Feb 13;209(2):211-5. doi: 10.1084/jem.20120162.
2. Zhao Y, Butler EB, Tan M. Targeting cellular metabolism to improve cancer therapeutics. Cell Death Dis. 2013 Mar 7;4:e532. doi: 10.1038/cddis.2013.60.
3. Kurtoglu M, Gao N, Shang J, Maher JC, Lehrman MA, Wangpaichitr M, Savaraj N, Lane AN, Lampidis TJ. Under normoxia, 2-deoxy-D-glucose elicits cell death in select tumor types not by inhibition of glycolysis but by interfering with N-linked glycosylation. Mol Cancer Ther. 2007 Nov;6(11):3049-58.
4. Gallamini A, Zwarthoed C, Borra A. Positron Emission Tomography (PET) in Oncology. Cancers (Basel). 2014 Dec; 6(4): 1821–1889.
5. Xi H, Kurtoglu M, Lampidis TJ. The wonders of 2-deoxy-D-glucose. IUBMB Life. 2014 Feb;66(2):110-21. doi: 10.1002/iub.1251.

Angiogenesis inhibitors, cutting off cancers' supply lines

Besides tricking cancer cells to take in glucose analogs to inhibit their glucose metabolism, another way to cut off their energy supply is through direct inhibition of blood vessels using a group of compounds called angiogenesis inhibitors. Cancer metastasis requires an increase in blood supply, through which they attain by generating new blood vessels, a process called angiogenesis. Although today this is a commonly used tactic, many leaders in the cancer field were skeptical when Dr. Folkman first presented the initially radical concept during the 1970s. However, when clinical trials began to prove the efficacy of this strategy, the FDA approved the first angiogenesis inhibitor Bevacizumab in treating colorectal cancer in 2004. Since then, Bevacizumab has been approved to treat of various other types of cancer including lung cancer, cervical cancer, breast cancer, and many more.

Angiogenesis is a tightly controlled process that is usually triggered by low oxygen levels in tissue. Rapid proliferation and metabolism of cancer cells generate areas in the tumor that have low oxygen levels. These conditions are known as hypoxic stress, which lead to the stabilization of a protein called hypoxia inducible factor-1α (HIF-1α). HIF-1α in turn upregulates a plethora of angiogenesis inducers, most important among them is the vascular endothelial growth factor (VEGF). VEGF is secreted by cancers under hypoxic stress, which then binds to its receptors (VEGFRs) on the membrane of endothelial cells. This leads to the proliferation of endothelial cells and thus the formation of new blood vessels. By using this strategy, cancer cells can redirect blood supply by inducing hypoxic stress, leading to tumor expansion and progression.

Each step involved in angiogenesis mentioned above can be targeted for inhibition of angiogenesis, which can shrink tumor volume. The first-in-class angiogenesis inhibitor Bevacizumab functions by specifically binding to VEGF to keep it from interacting with its receptor

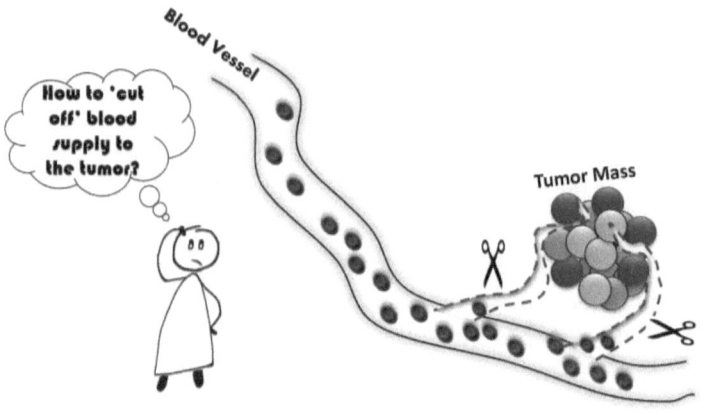

Figure 2.2: Cutting off blood supply to the tumor mass can curb tumor growth. This process can be accomplished surgically by directly cutting off blood vessels or by using angiogenesis inhibitors.

VEGFR. Another strategy to target VEGF is using Aflibercept (VEGF-trap), which contains a portion of the VEGF receptor that is responsible for the interaction between VEGF and VEGFR. Consequently, Aflibercept can "trap" VEGF by binding to its VEGFR binding sites, occluding its interaction with the VEGFR. Aflibercept is approved for the treatment of colorectal cancer and multiple clinical trials are currently taking place to evaluate its efficacy in other types of tumors. Do you have any other ideas that may work in keeping VEGF from binding VEGFR? Write it down as it may become another brand-new antitumor strategy!

Direct inhibition of VEGFR has also been studied that lead to the discovery of broad spectrum tyrosine kinase inhibitors (TKIs) including Sunitinib, Sorafenib and Erlotinib that actively inhibit VEGFR activation/phosphorylation. Upon binding with its ligands, VEGFR dimerizes and autophosphorylates, setting off a chain of downstream signaling pathways that promote endothelial cell growth and division. Consequently, TKIs that are active against EGFR, another group of cancer-related cell receptors, are also being studied as VEGFR inhibitors to inhibit angiogenesis. Humanized antibodies that can directly eradicate the activation of VEGFR are still under development, with some promising preclinical data that has just been reported recently.

Is inhibition of angiogenesis an effective strategy for the treatment of hematopoietic cancers like leukemia? Why?

Reference

1. Folkman J. Tumor angiogenesis: therapeutic implications. N Engl J Med. 1971 Nov 18;285(21):1182-6.
2. Kim KJ, Li B, Winer J, Armanini M, Gillett N, Phillips HS, Ferrara N. Inhibition of vascular endothelial growth factor-induced angiogenesis suppresses tumour growth in vivo. Nature. 1993 Apr 29;362(6423):841-4.
3. Holash J, Davis S, Papadopoulos N, Croll SD, Ho L, Russell M, Boland P, Leidich R, Hylton D, Burova E, Ioffe E, Huang T, Radziejewski C, Bailey K, Fandl JP, Daly T, Wiegand SJ, Yancopoulos GD, Rudge JS. VEGF-Trap: a VEGF blocker with potent antitumor effects. Proc Natl Acad Sci U S A. 2002 Aug 20;99(17):11393-8.
4. Cook KM, Figg WD. Angiogenesis inhibitors: current strategies and future prospects. CA Cancer J Clin. 2010 Jul-Aug;60(4):222-43.
5. El-Kenawi AE, El-Remessy AB. Angiogenesis inhibitors in cancer therapy: mechanistic perspective on classification and treatment rationales. Br J Pharmacol. 2013 Oct;170(4):712-29.
6. Morabito A, De Maio E, Di Maio M, Normanno N, Perrone F. Tyrosine kinase inhibitors of vascular endothelial growth factor receptors in clinical trials: current status and future directions. Oncologist. 2006 Jul-Aug;11(7):753-64.
7. Atzori MG, Tentori L, Ruffini F, Ceci C, Lisi L, Bonanno E, Scimeca M, Eskilsson E, Daubon T, Miletic H, Ricci Vitiani L, Pallini R, Navarra P, Bjerkvig R, D'Atri S, Lacal PM, Graziani G. The anti-vascular endothelial growth factor receptor-1 monoclonal antibody D16F7 inhibits invasiveness of human glioblastoma and glioblastoma stem cells. J Exp Clin Cancer Res. 2017 Aug 10;36(1):106.

Chicken or the Egg: IDH mutations and Tumorigenesis

Almost one century after the discovery of the 'Warburg' effect, we are still at the rudimentary stage of understanding the underlying genetic alterations responsible for this occurrence. The general consensus was that cancer cells shut off the function of mitochondria to redirect the intermediates generated by glucose metabolism towards of cell structure integrity. Recent studies now indicate that shutting down mitochondria surprisingly help fuel the energy consumption of cancer cells by promoting angiogenesis. This phenomenon is more pronounced in cancer cells that harbor isocitrate dehydrogenase (IDH) mutations.

IDHs are a group of enzymes that mainly function in mitochondria to convert isocitrate into α-ketoglutarate (α-KG), CO_2, and anti-oxidant NADPH. This process is one of the steps of the famous TCA cycle that is responsible for metabolizing glucose into CO_2, energy (ATP), and heat. In certain tumor types such as Glioblastoma multiforme (GBM), acute myeloid leukemia (AML), and chondrosarcomas, IDH is often mutated, causing a near complete shutdown of mitochondrial function. Mutated IDH instead converts isocitrate into 2-hydroxyglutarate (2-HG), which cannot be further metabolized in the mitochondria for energy production. This mutation not only shuts down the TCA cycle but also decreases the cellular concentration of NADPH. Counterintuitively, because NADPH is an important anti-oxidant, glioma patients harboring IDH mutations generally have better prognosis post chemotherapy and radiotherapy. On the other hand, mutated IDH leads to decreased concentrations of α-KG, which degrades hypoxia inducible factor-1α (HIF-1α), a critical factor that can induce angiogenesis. Depletion of α-KG promotes longevity of HIF-1α, thus upregulating angiogenesis.

The accumulation of 2-HG plays vital roles in promoting tumor progression. It is now well-demonstrated that a surplus of 2-HG in IDH-mutated cancer cells can inhibit DNA demethylase, leading to

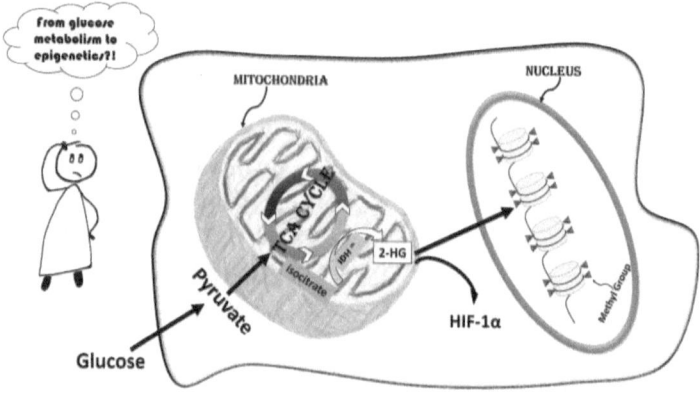

Figure 2.4: Some types of cancer has mutated IDHs. Mutated forms of IDHs will impede normal glucose metabolism. Meanwhile, they can produce 2HG, which will upregulate HIF-1α and DNA methylation, both of which will promote tumor progression.

DNA hypermethylation. As previously discussed, DNA hypermethylation prevents the transcription of tumor suppressors and differentiation-inducing genes, which leads to uninhibited growth of malignant cells. Due to its oncogenic effects, 2-HG is now called an 'oncometabolite' – a metabolic intermediate that causes tumor. Because high levels of 2-HG are usually only detected in patients with IDH mutations, physicians can utilize serum levels of 2-HG of their patients to assess their prognosis.

Let us recap the significance of IDH mutations. IDH mutations shut down mitochondria, causing cells to become almost completely dependent on glycolysis for ATP generation. Intermediates generated from glycolysis provide building blocks for cell proliferation. Resultant 2-HG induces angiogenesis to redirect glucose to fuel transformed cancer cells. More significantly, 2-HG also modifies our DNA by suppressing guards that normally protect healthy cells from malignant transformation.

Every new breakthrough allows us to get closer to discovering the "Achilles heel" of cancer. In 2017, Idhifa (enasidenib) was approved by FDA as the first IDH inhibitor for the treatment of relapsed or refractory AML. Since the first report of IDH mutations in glioma in 2009 and the recent approval of its clinical inhibitor Idhifa, scientists and clinicians have brought new hopes for patients with deteriorating types of cancer.

Reference
1. Zhao S, Lin Y, Xu W, Jiang W, Zha Z, Wang P, Yu W, Li Z, Gong L, Peng Y, Ding J, Lei Q, Guan KL, Xiong Y. Glioma-derived mutations in IDH1 dominantly inhibit IDH1 catalytic activity and induce HIF-1alpha. Science. 2009 Apr 10;324(5924):261-5.
2. Yang H, Ye D, Guan KL, Xiong Y. IDH1 and IDH2 mutations in tumorigenesis: mechanistic insights and clinical perspectives. Clin Cancer Res. 2012 Oct 15;18(20):5562-71.
3. Xu W, Yang H, Liu Y, Yang Y, Wang P, Kim SH, Ito S, Yang C, Wang P, Xiao MT, Liu LX, Jiang WQ, Liu

J, Zhang JY, Wang B, Frye S, Zhang Y, Xu YH, Lei QY, Guan KL, Zhao SM, Xiong Y. Oncometabolite 2-hydroxyglutarate is a competitive inhibitor of α-ketoglutarate-dependent dioxygenases. Cancer Cell. 2011 Jan 18;19(1):17-30.

4. Chowdhury R, Yeoh KK, Tian YM, Hillringhaus L, Bagg EA, Rose NR, Leung IK, Li XS, Woon EC, Yang M, McDonough MA, King ON, Clifton IJ, Klose RJ, Claridge TD, Ratcliffe PJ, Schofield CJ, Kawamura A. The oncometabolite 2-hydroxyglutarate inhibits histone lysine demethylases. EMBO Rep. 2011 May;12(5):463-9.

5. Lu C, Ward PS, Kapoor GS, Rohle D, Turcan S, Abdel-Wahab O, Edwards CR, Khanin R, Figueroa ME, Melnick A, Wellen KE, O'Rourke DM, Berger SL, Chan TA, Levine RL, Mellinghoff IK, Thompson CB. IDH mutation impairs histone demethylation and results in a block to cell differentiation. Nature. 2012 Feb 15;483(7390):474-8.

6. Fathi AT, DiNardo CD, Kline I, Kenvin L, Gupta I, Attar EC, Stein EM, de Botton S; AG221-C-001 Study Investigators. Differentiation Syndrome Associated With Enasidenib, a Selective Inhibitor of Mutant Isocitrate Dehydrogenase 2: Analysis of a Phase 1/2 Study. JAMA Oncol. 2018 Jan 18.

7. DiNardo CD, Propert KJ, Loren AW, Paietta E, Sun Z, Levine RL, Straley KS, Yen K, Patel JP, Agresta S, Abdel-Wahab O, Perl AE, Litzow MR, Rowe JM, Lazarus HM, Fernandez HF, Margolis DJ, Tallman MS, Luger SM, Carroll M. Serum 2-hydroxyglutarate levels predict isocitrate dehydrogenase mutations and clinical outcome in acute myeloid leukemia. Blood. 2013 Jun 13;121(24):4917-24.

Depriving cancer of essential amino acids

Amino acids are the building blocks that cells use to make proteins. While healthy cells are capable of independently synthesizing their own asparagine, arginine and glutamine, some types of cancer cells are dependent on obtaining these key amino acids from our diet instead. The metabolic reprograming that occurs in cancer cells partially contributes to tumor progression by shutting down certain enzymes required for the synthesis of these nonessential amino acids. Because of the rapid replication rate that cancer cells undergo, they require sustained synthesis of new proteins to make new copies of themselves. As a result, deprivation of these amino acids that are required for tumor growth will halt protein synthesis and lead to apoptosis, whereas healthy cells still have the enzymes to make those amino acids and thus can survive without them.

Guided by these thinking, several strategies were developed in depriving these amino acids to slow down tumor growth. Ideally, complete cut off of these amino acids from diet will have anti-tumor effects as has been proven in preclinical conditions. In clinic, however, these amino acids are deprived from blood circulation by using corresponding enzymes that can specifically convert an amino acid to another compound that tumor cells cannot use while healthy cells are able to convert it back to the original amino acid once absorbed.

While most compounds that target amino acid depletion for cancer therapy are still under clinical trials, deprivation of asparagine using L-asparaginase has been used to treat acute lymphoblastic leukemia for almost five decades. L-asparaginase, derived from E. coli, can convert

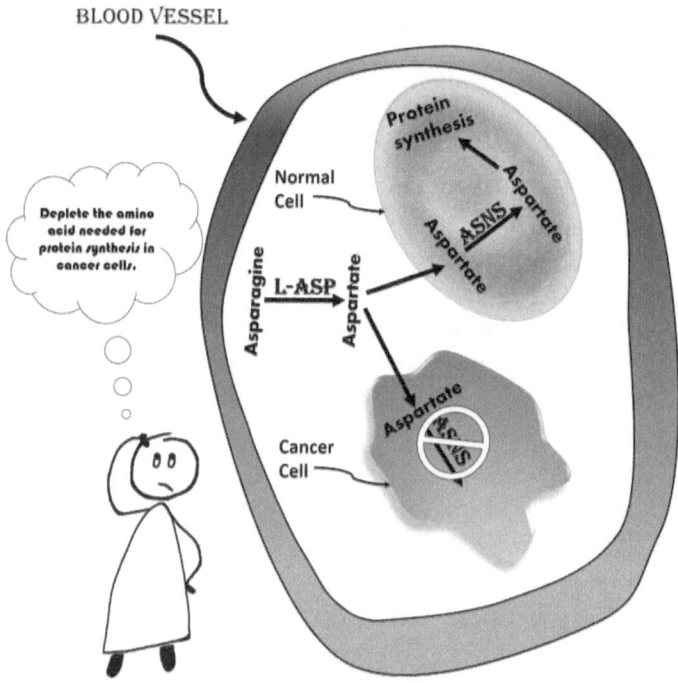

Figure 2.5: Enzymes like L-asparaginase (L-ASP) can deplete amino acids that cancer cells are dependent on for protein synthesis. Normal tissue cells can overcome L-ASP-mediated depletion of asparagine since it express asparagine synthetase (ASNS). Cancer cells lost the ASNS expression and thus cannot regenerate asparaginase from aspartate, leading to inhibition of protein synthesis and cause cell death.

asparagine to aspartate which can be converted back to asparagine once absorbed in healthy tissue cells. Cancer cells lack this essential enzyme that is responsible for the conversion. This drug-induced asparagine starvation stops protein synthesis and interrupts protein folding in cancer cells, leading to apoptosis.

However, cancer cells may develop resistance mechanisms to L-asparaginase treatment which causes cancer relapse. In addition, because L-asparaginase is a "foreign" protein derived from bacteria, our own bodies may develop antibodies to deactivate L-asparaginase, leading to regrowth of cancer cells. Other amino acids can also be targets for deprivation. For example, arginine deaminase can induce arginine starvation by converting arginine to citrulline, a compound cannot be reconverted back to arginine in certain cancers. Also, another recent drug called Arginase I can convert arginine to ornithine, which is unusable for protein synthesis in certain cancers. These studies broadened the types of cancer that can be treated by amino acid deprivation.

Interestingly, dietary restriction of amino acids in curbing tumor suppression is controversial. Recent studies using animal models with intestinal cancer or lymphoma were deprived of serine and glycine via diet restriction showed promising results in controlling tumor growth. However, in vivo trials have yet to reciprocate the same successful results so please do not use this as a therapeutic suggestion for cancer treatment.

A more straightforward but not as selective mechanism to inhibit protein synthesis is to directly shut down protein synthesis. This strategy has shown to effectively wipe out cancer cells cultured in petri dishes. For example, the anti-tumor effects of both popular chemotherapeutic agents dactinomycin and bleomycin are partly attributed to their capacity in inhibiting protein synthesis. However, since protein synthesis is also essential for the survival of normal cells, protein synthesis inhibitors usually come with deleterious side effects when used in treating cancer patients.

Reference
1. Maddocks ODK, Athineos D, Cheung EC, Lee P, Zhang T, van den Broek NJF, Mackay GM, Labuschagne CF, Gay D1, Kruiswijk F, Blagih J, Vincent DF, Campbell KJ, Ceteci F, Sansom OJ, Blyth K, Vousden KH. Modulating the therapeutic response of tumours to dietary serine and glycine starvation. Nature. 2017 Apr 19;544(7650):372-376.
2. Tsai HJ, Jiang SS, Hung WC, Borthakur G, Lin SF, Pemmaraju N, Jabbour E, Bomalaski JS, Chen YP, Hsiao HH, Wang MC, Kuo CY, Chang H, Yeh SP, Cortes J, Chen LT, Chen TY. A Phase II Study of Arginine Deiminase (ADI-PEG20) in Relapsed/Refractory or Poor-Risk Acute Myeloid Leukemia Patients. Sci Rep. 2017 Sep 12;7(1):11253.
3. Fung MKL, Chan GC. Drug-induced amino acid deprivation as strategy for cancer therapy. J Hematol Oncol. 2017 Jul 27;10(1):144.
4. Patel N, Krishnan S, Offman MN, Krol M, Moss CX, Leighton C, van Delft FW, Holland M, Liu J, Alexander S, Dempsey C, Ariffin H, Essink M, Eden TO, Watts C, Bates PA, Saha V. A dyad of lymphoblastic lysosomal cysteine proteases degrades the antileukemic drug L-asparaginase. J Clin Invest. 2009 Jul;119(7):1964-73.
5. Abraham AT, Lin JJ, Newton DL, Rybak S, Hecht SM. RNA cleavage and inhibition of protein synthesis by bleomycin. Chem Biol. 2003 Jan;10(1):45-52.
6. Cuyàs E, Martin-Castillo B, Corominas-Faja B, Massaguer A, Bosch-Barrera J, Menendez JA. Anti-protozoal and anti-bacterial antibiotics that inhibit protein synthesis kill cancer subtypes enriched for stem cell-like properties. Cell Cycle. 2015;14(22):3527-32.

Shuhua (Steve) Zheng, Ph.D.

Shutting down the recycling center via proteasome inhibition

While protein synthesis is essential for cell survival, timely degradation of surplus or damaged proteins are equally, if not more, important in keeping cells viable. Protein synthesis is similar to the production of vehicles, tools, and utensils that we purchase to expedite activities in our own lives. When these items break or no longer have use, we need to recycle them. Otherwise, our community will be brimming with trash and will ultimately become unsustainable. In cells, the accumulation of damaged or unnecessary proteins will not only make them "crowded", but also cause them to become cytotoxic. This recycling process is essential for the survival of both malignant and health cells.

Cancer cells require faster protein turnover to constantly generate new "tools" to be utilized in different stages of proliferation. In slow-cycling healthy cells, a single tool set can sustain cell survival for a much longer period of time. Based on this idea, therapeutic agents have been developed to specifically shut down these protein degradation machineries.

Protein degradation is mainly carried out by a highly regulated process called ubiquitin-proteasome system (UPS) to ensure only unnecessary/damaged proteins are marked for destruction. First, a small peptide protein called ubiquitin is tagged to proteins that need to be degraded. This causes a cascade of more ubiquitin proteins to attach to the first ubiquitin, forming a ubiquitin chain. This ubiquitin chain guides the dysfunctional protein to a large complex responsible for the destruction process itself called the proteasome.

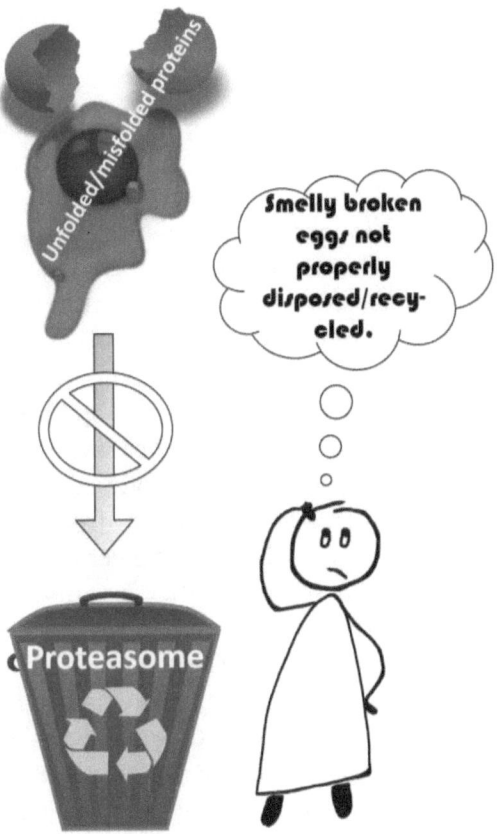

Figure 2.6: Proteasome is the major cell machinery responsible for protein degradation. Inhibition of proteasome will promote accumulated of misfolded, dysfunctional proteins. Accumulation of these proteins will impede protein cycling and cause cell death.

These dysfunctional proteins are recycled into reusable amino acids at the end of proteasome-mediated degradation.

The first generation of compounds that target this pathway by directly inhibiting proteasomes include bortezomib, carfilzomib and ixazomib and are used mainly for the treatment of multiple myeloma and other types of cancer. These drugs cause the accumulation of surplus and damaged proteins, which trigger cytotoxic effects mainly via a process called endoplasmic reticulum (ER) stress. The ER is the site of protein synthesis in cells that generate crude proteins and help modify them to carry out their required functions once released from the ER. Proteins that are not properly modified in the ER are tagged by ubiquitins and discharged from ER to be degraded by proteasomes. Because cancer cells undergo a faster rate of protein synthesis, they are more prone to producing dysfunctional proteins than healthy tissue cells. When proteasomes are blocked by drugs such as bortezomib, these dysfunctional proteins accumulate in the ER and overwhelm the ER. Some types of cancer cells are especially sensitive to ER stress.

Besides triggering ER stress, another major cytotoxic mechanism of proteasome inhibitors is the inhibition of pro-survival pathways, especially through the notorious nuclear factor kB (NF-kB) pathway. The inhibitor of this pathway, called IκBα, needs to be constantly degraded by the UPS to keep this pro-survival pathway and allow the progression of several tumor types. Inhibition of the proteasome, allows IκBα to accumulate and further inhibit the NF-kB pathway, leading to cancer cell death. Because malignant cells are usually more dependent on the NF-kB pathway, proteasome inhibition has a higher sensitivity in targeting cancer cells.

Reference
1. Shen M, Schmitt S, Buac D, Dou QP. Targeting the ubiquitin-proteasome system for cancer therapy. Expert Opin Ther Targets. 2013 Sep;17(9):1091-108.
2. Manasanch EE, Orlowski RZ. Proteasome inhibitors in cancer therapy. Nat Rev Clin Oncol. 2017 Jul;14(7):417-433
3. Orlowski RZ, Kuhn DJ. Proteasome inhibitors in cancer therapy: lessons from the first decade. Clin Cancer Res. 2008 Mar 15;14(6):1649-57
4. Hanke NT, Garland LL, Baker AF. Carfilzomib combined with suberanilohydroxamic acid (SAHA) synergistically promotes endoplasmic reticulum stress in non-small cell lung cancer cell lines. J Cancer Res Clin Oncol. 2016 Mar;142(3):549-60.
5. Cusack JC. Rationale for the treatment of solid tumors with the proteasome inhibitor bortezomib. Cancer Treat Rev. 2003 May;29 Suppl 1:21-31.

CHAPTER III: PUSH FOR DIFFERENTIATION

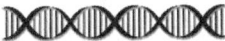

"It is proposed that most neoplasms arise from a single cell of origin, and tumor progression results from acquired genetic variability within the original clone allowing sequential selection of more aggressive sublines."

Peter Nowell, M.D.

"Some aspects of tumor development resemble processes seen in developing organs, whereas others are more akin to tissue remodeling."

Mikala Egeblad, Ph.D.

"Well-differentiated cancer cells look more like normal cells and tend to grow and spread more slowly than poorly differentiated or undifferentiated cancer cells"

National Cancer Institute

"But if they do (existence of cancer stem cells), there is going to be a paradigm shift in the way that chemotherapy efficacy is evaluated and how therapeutics are developed."

Luis Parada, Ph.D.

Shuhua (Steve) Zheng, Ph.D.

Introduction

In the 1970s, Dr. Nowell proposed that cancer arises from a single cell of origin that has accumulated genetic alterations. Now, after more than four decades of research, we finally have enough evidence to support his conjecture. Darwin's theory of evolution, "the survival of the fittest", explains the selection process of a single cell that gives rise to a whole tumor. Tissue cells can randomly acquire genetic alterations due to defects in DNA replication or radiation. Fortunately, in most cases, these DNA alterations are harmless. Cells that have acquired extensive mutations undergo apoptosis by our immune system. However, cells that survive this strict selection process gain the opportunity to give rise to a tumor. It is a common misconception that this selected cancerous cell performs clonal replication to create the mass of a tumor. Instead, a tumor mass is more like an organ, consisting of a plethora of different types of cells. The question is, how does a single cancerous cell give rise to such a heterogenous population of cancer cells in a tumor mass?

The story starts with a single selected cell resembling a stem cell that gives rise to a tumor. As you may know, the integrity of a functional tissue or organ is maintained by stem cells that stay quiescent for most of the time. Their replication is triggered when replacement of tissue cells is required, generating another stem cell for self-renewal and a differentiated cell for replacement. Scientists believe the process of self-renewal and differentiation also happen during tumorigenesis in that one single selected cancer cell generates a tumor mass that consists of many different cell types. These tumorigenic cells that give rise to a tumor are now called cancer stem cells (CSCs). Their

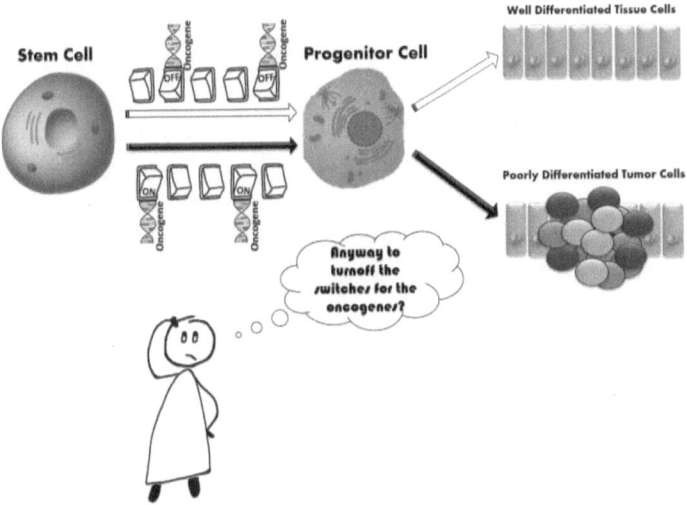

Figure 3.1: Due to activation of oncogenes or other unknown events, the normal differentiation of cells can be inhibited. This process can generate poorly differentiated malignant cells that are often more difficult to treat.

discovery has many significant therapeutic implications for cancer management discussed in more details in this chapter.

While the offspring of normal stem cells generate differentiated cells that integrate into tissues and organs to maintain functionality, most descendants of CSCs are poorly differentiated, fast-replicating cells that constitute the majority of a tumor mass. Clinical grading of tumors is heavily dependent on the differentiation status of the cancer cells in the mass. A tumor with poorly differentiated cancer cells usually receives the worst grading because the cells replicate faster and are more prone to undergo metastasis than relatively well-differentiated cancer cells. Scientists have discovered ways to induce differentiation in cancer cells to curb their proliferation and progression.

Because the discovery of CSCs in tumors is quite recent, there are many questions still left unanswered. In this chapter, we will introduce well-established strategies that target poorly differentiated cancer cells. With more research, we hope to see more approaches and drugs that target this feature of cancer.

Reference
1. Nowell PC. The clonal evolution of tumor cell populations. Science. 1976 Oct 1;194(4260):23-8.
2. Egeblad M, Nakasone ES, Werb Z. Tumors as organs: complex tissues that interface with the entire organism. Dev Cell. 2010 Jun 15;18(6):884-901.
3. Plaks V, Kong N, Werb Z. The cancer stem cell niche: how essential is the niche in regulating stemness of tumor cells? Cell Stem Cell. 2015 Mar 5;16(3):225-38.
4. Adam JK, Odhav B, Bhoola KD. Immune responses in cancer. Pharmacol Ther. 2003 Jul;99(1):113-32.

Pushing cancer cells back to its differentiated status

Healthy tissue cells are usually derived from normal progenitor cells that can divide and self-renew. The population of these progenitor cells decreases as we become older and as a result, our tissue cells no longer readily replace themselves and aging occurs. On the other hand, cancer cells avoid "aging" by reversing the process of differentiation. By doing so, cancer cells transform from well-differentiated tissues back into a progenitor-like state to regain the ability to divide and self-renew. This tumorigenic process is often termed 'dedifferentiation'.

Given the similarity of the molecular features of cancer cells with normal progenitor cells, some scientists call cancer a developmental disease. The story of the dedifferentiation in cancer cells is even more complicated by the recent discovery of CSCs. In a clinical setting, the differentiation status of cancer cells is monitored using biomarkers to help determine the stage of the tumor. In this section, we will focus on how poorly-differentiated cancer cells can be pharmaceutically forced to differentiate thus inhibiting cancer progression.

The most popular differentiation-inducing agent is retinoic acid (RA) which is also essential for normal embryo development. When RA binds to retinoic acid receptors (RARs) inside cells, it triggers a cascade of events that cause the binding of RARs to specific genomic regions that transcriptionally regulate differentiation-inducing gene expression. However, as mentioned in the previous story, the promoter regions of tumor suppressors are often inaccessible due to HDAC-mediated deacetylation. This is why activated RARS may still be unable to access their target genes, giving rise to

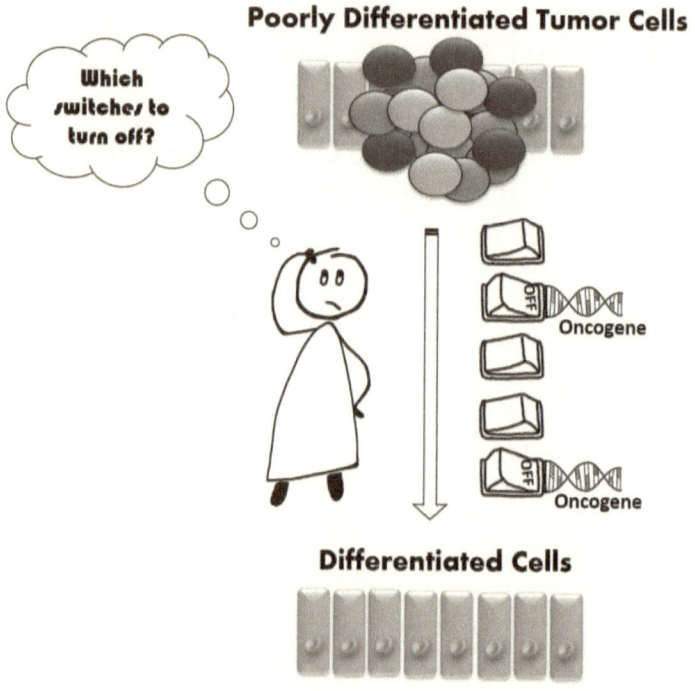

Figure 3.2: Some types of the poorly differentiated cancer cells can be treated with differentiate-inducing agents. Also, inhibition of oncogenes and/or upregulating of tumor suppressor genes can also promote the fully differentiation of cells.

resistance developed from RA treatment alone in the clinical setting. Addition of HDAC inhibitors induce DNA to become more susceptible to the binding of RARs, and in turn upregulates expression of genes that promote cancer cell differentiation.

Interestingly, one of the most potent differentiation-inducing agent used in practice is arsenic trioxide, an ancient toxic compound used as a therapeutic agent for more than 2000 years. In the 1990s, clinical trials that took place in China showed that treatments using arsenic trioxide alone induced 70% to 90% complete remission in patients that were newly diagnosed with acute promyelocytic leukemia (APL). Since then, arsenic trioxide is used globally as the frontline treatment of choice for APL. The mechanism of action for arsenic trioxide is through inducing RARs activation and oxidative stress. Given that most healthy tissue cells are already terminally differentiated, arsenic trioxide treatment has minimal side effects if treatment regimen is strictly adhered to.

You might wonder, if RA is a derivative of vitamin A (retinol), can vitamin A supplements prevent cancer? Unfortunately, there is a lack of solid clinical trials that can definitely answer this question. Furthermore, one comprehensive overview showed there was no evidence of vitamin A preventing or treating lung cancer. And of course, it is well-documented that over-doses of vitamin A supplements can cause liver damage, severe nausea and headaches, etc.

Reference

1. de Thé H. Differentiation therapy revisited. Nat Rev Cancer. 2018 Feb;18(2):117-127. doi: 10.1038/nrc.2017.103. Epub 2017 Dec 1.
2. Kawamata H, Tachibana M, Fujimori T, Imai Y. Differentiation-inducing therapy for solid tumors. Curr Pharm Des. 2006;12(3):379-85.
3. Zhu J, Chen Z, Lallemand-Breitenbach V, de Thé H. How acute promyelocytic leukaemia revived arsenic. Nat Rev Cancer. 2002 Sep;2(9):705-13.
4. Tang XH, Gudas LJ. Retinoids, retinoic acid receptors, and cancer. Annu Rev Pathol. 2011;6:345-64.
5. Pili R, Salumbides B, Zhao M, Altiok S, Qian D, Zwiebel J, Carducci MA, Rudek MA. Phase I study of the histone deacetylase inhibitor entinostat in combination with 13-cis retinoic acid in patients with solid tumours. Br J Cancer. 2012 Jan 3;106(1):77-84.
6. Fritz H, Kennedy D, Fergusson D, Fernandes R, Doucette S, Cooley K, Seely A, Sagar S, Wong R, Seely D. Vitamin A and retinoid derivatives for lung cancer: a systematic review and meta analysis. PLoS One. 2011;6(6):e21107.

Eradicating cancer stem cells, how to get there

In addition to the theory that cancer is a developmental disease, scientists proposed that a tumor is an abnormal organ consisting of cells with various differentiated states and functions. To further prove this idea, scientists have identified a small population of cells within tumors that are slow-cycling but are self-renewing and can differentiate into different lineages like normal tissue stem cells. Tumors were initially seen as masses composed of solely fast-replicating cells. This idea was challenged by the discovery of the small subgroup of cancer cells called cancer stem cells (CSCs). Considering the fact that a single embryonic stem cell can generate an entire human body, CSCs can also generate an entire tumor from a single cancer cell in theory whereas fast-replicating cancer cells often do not.

Since most chemotherapies only target fast-replicating cancer cells, it is very unlikely that slow-replicating CSCs are killed during traditional therapy, leading to drug resistance and relapse. Initial treatments shrink tumors by killing fast-replicating cancer cells whereas CSCs often survive the chemotherapy and in turn generate cancer cells with resistance. Because only CSCs can form new tumors, dissemination of CSCs from a primary tumor is responsible for tumor metastasis. Increased levels of cancer cells with stem cell like features in circulation often indicate poor prognosis. Furthermore, CSCs were identified as being responsible for the generation of endothelia cells involved in angiogenesis during tumor progression.

If we can eradicate progenitor cancer cells, tumors will be less prone to developing resistance, relapse and

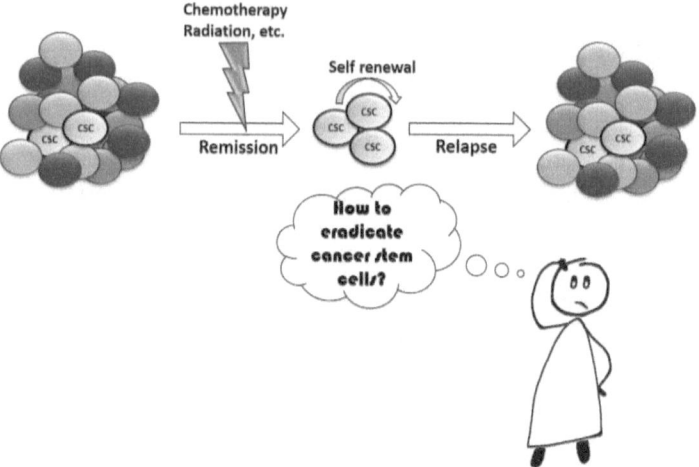

Figure 3.3: Cancer stem cells (CSCs) are a group of malignant cells that have features similar to normal tissue stem cells. These cells are often resistant to treatment. They are believed to be responsible for relapse after remission.

metastasis as well. So how can we kill CSCs? While there has been tremendous progress in identifying of CSCs in last decade, therapeutic targeting of CSCs is still in its rudimentary stage. To maintain its self-renewal abilities, CSCs need to reactivate pathways that are usually turned off after the early steps of human embryo development. For example, the reactivation of the Notch, Wnt/beta-catenin, and Hedgehog signaling pathway were shown to being critical in maintaining self-renewal and pluripotency (ability to differentiate into different lineages of cells) of CSCs. However, scientists have yet to uncover whether reactivation of Hedgehog, Wnt and Notch is involved in the initial generation of CSCs.

Inhibition of these pathways has been proven to be a

difficult task. First and foremast, only Hedgehog inhibitor, Vismodegib, has been approved by the FDA in treating metastatic basal cell carcinoma. Laboratory studies have also shown depletion of CSCs with its use, bringing hope for a new generation of therapeutic regimens that have lower chances of relapsing. In addition, celecoxib, which is already used in practice for the treatment of arthritis and was initially studied as a Wnt pathway inhibitor, has received FDA approval for the prevention of colorectal cancer.

Reference
1. Egeblad M, Nakasone ES, Werb Z. Tumors as organs: complex tissues that interface with the entire organism. Dev Cell. 2010 Jun 15;18(6):884-901.
2. Friedmann-Morvinski D, Verma IM. Dedifferentiation and reprogramming: origins of cancer stem cells. EMBO Rep. 2014 Mar;15(3):244-53.
3. Ping YF, Bian XW. Consice review: Contribution of cancer stem cells to neovascularization. Stem Cells. 2011 Jun;29(6):888-94.
4. Rycaj K, Tang DG. Cell-of-Origin of Cancer versus Cancer Stem Cells: Assays and Interpretations. Cancer Res. 2015 Oct 1;75(19):4003-11.
5. Takebe N, Miele L, Harris PJ, Jeong W, Bando H, Kahn M, Yang SX, Ivy SP. Targeting Notch, Hedgehog, and Wnt pathways in cancer stem cells: clinical update. Nat Rev Clin Oncol. 2015 Aug;12(8):445-64.
6. Takahashi K, Tanabe K, Ohnuki M, Narita M, Ichisaka T, Tomoda K, Yamanaka S. Induction of pluripotent stem cells from adult human fibroblasts by defined factors. Cell. 2007 Nov 30;131(5):861-72.

7. Kelly KF, Ng DY, Jayakumaran G, Wood GA, Koide H, Doble BW. β-catenin enhances Oct-4 activity and reinforces pluripotency through a TCF-independent mechanism. Cell Stem Cell. 2011 Feb 4;8(2):214-27.
8. Singh BN, Fu J, Srivastava RK, Shankar S. Hedgehog signaling antagonist GDC-0449 (Vismodegib) inhibits pancreatic cancer stem cell characteristics: molecular mechanisms. PLoS One. 2011;6(11):e27306.
9. Sotiropoulou PA, Christodoulou MS, Silvani A, Herold-Mende C, Passarella D. Chemical approaches to targeting drug resistance in cancer stem cells. Drug Discov Today. 2014 Oct;19(10):1547-62.

Shuhua (Steve) Zheng, Ph.D.

CHAPTER IV: TARGETED THERAPY

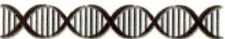

"For a lot of people, Gleevec was simply too good to be true. But these once-dying patients were getting out of bed, dancing, going hiking, doing yoga. The drug was amazing."

Brian J. Druker, M.D.

"... the effect (of targeted TKI therapy) was almost immediate. Two weeks later, his bone marrow aspirate showed that Harrison was in remission – no signs of the cancer!"

Steve McKinion, a cancer-survivor's father

"... it became apparent that targeted cancer therapy(TCT) actions do not restrict themselves to tumour cells, and TCT is not without adverse effects or complications."

Dale Lee Bixby, M.D., Ph.D.

"... the average insurance payment per month for targeted oral therapies has skyrocketed, from just over $3000 a month to $7000 in a 10-year period."

Fabrice Smieliauskas, Ph.D.

Introduction

As the author of this book, I am happy to personally introduce you to this chapter. Targeted therapy has made many long-awaited medical miracles in the field of cancer treatment that have never been seen before in medical history. The story begins with the advent and later worldwide usage of the first targeted therapy imatinib (Gleevec), that was developed in the 1990s to be used as treatment for cancer patients harboring the 'Philadelphia chromosome'. Since then, targeted therapies have been developed for many other types of cancer derived from mutated genes that drive tumor progression. As compared with traditional chemotherapy, targeted therapy spares healthy cells because their targets often only solely exist in cancer cells. This leads to a much reduced toxicity for patients. The principle behind targeted therapy is to alter one or more proteins that drive tumor progression to eradicate their functionality, which leads to remission. Thus, finding the right targets is critical in ensuring therapeutic efficacy.

From a molecular level, a cascade of proteins relays a cellular stimulus to facilitate the execution of a desired result. In healthy tissue cells, cell-signaling pathways are strictly regulated to ensure activation is only triggered when needed. However in cancer cells, their mutations generate proteins that cannot be turned off by negative regulatory mechanisms. As a result, specific signaling pathways are constantly active even in the absence of a stimulus.

Targeted therapy has made great strides in last two decades through significant technological achievements, such as in DNA sequencing, computer programing, and detailed molecular-level understanding of the events that

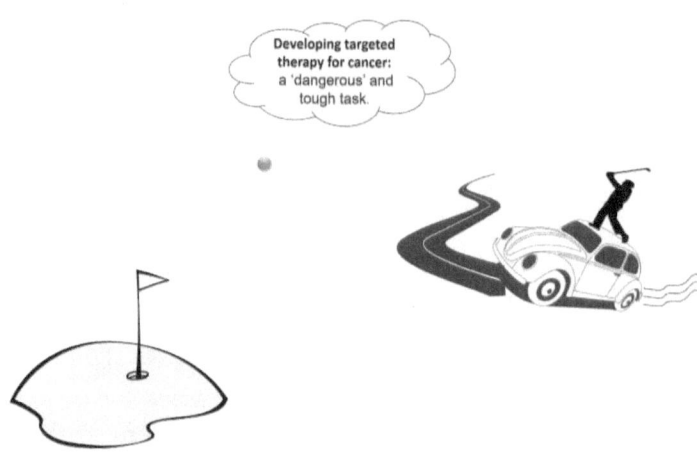

Figure 4.1: Development of a targeted therapy for cancer treatment involves tremendous investment. Years of laboratory and clinical studies are always required to guarantee the safety and efficacy of the newly developed targeted therapeutic agent.

occur during tumor progression. Development of targeted therapy begins with the identification of altered proteins caused by cancer cells, followed by biochemical studies and computer models that analyze the functional and structural dysfunctions. Based on the results, compounds that may be capable of inhibiting the mutated proteins are screened and selected for further study in both laboratory and clinical settings.

The process of identification and running functional tests are often time consuming and require significant financial investment. Unfortunately, even with the best screening and preclinical studies, most chosen compounds fail to replicate the same success during clinical trials. In fact, we are lucky to come across the few compounds that survive this rigorous process to ensure not only the efficacy but also more importantly, the safety of the patient. Although this is an overly simplified explanation of the timeline and tremendous investment that occurs in targeted therapy research, it may partly explain why these treatment options are often criticized for their cost.

However, targeted therapy is still far from perfect. They come with inherent disadvantages because they are designed to target highly specific binding sites on proteins that arise from mutations. Should these targeted therapy-binding sites become altered by further mutations, the drug itself becomes defective and obsolete. As we mentioned previously, the innate genomic instability of tumor cells causes them to be prone to subsequent DNA mutations. Under the stress of targeted therapy treatment, cancer cells that already harbor mutations can undergo further changes that modify the structure of a targeted protein or even activate an alternative protein that help the tumor develop resistance against the therapy.

Today, multiple drugs are often prescribed together that not only target the same protein but also different mutations. Relapse or loss of sensitivity to the treatment often calls for genetic testing to reveal secondary mutations to administer corresponding targeted therapies. We hope after reading this chapter, you will have an overview of how targeted therapies are designed and how key components in signaling pathways are chosen to be targets for treatment.

Reference

1. Iqbal N, Iqbal N. Imatinib: a breakthrough of targeted therapy in cancer. Chemother Res Pract. 2014;2014:357027.
2. Druker BJ. Perspectives on the development of a molecularly targeted agent. Cancer Cell. 2002 Feb;1(1):31-6.
3. Helwick C. Researchers Dissect the Cost of Targeted Agents. Am Health Drug Benefits. 2015 Aug;8(Spec Issue):10.
4. Ellis LM, Hicklin DJ. Resistance to Targeted Therapies: Refining Anticancer Therapy in the Era of Molecular Oncology. Clin Cancer Res. 2009 Dec 15;15(24):7471-7478.
5. Talati C, Pinilla-Ibarz J. Resistance in chronic myeloid leukemia: definitions and novel therapeutic agents. Curr Opin Hematol. 2018 Mar;25(2):154-161.

Imatinib (Gleevec) - A paradigm shift in cancer therapy

While efficient in inducing cancer cell death, traditional chemotherapy usually cannot differentiate between normal cells from malignant ones as discussed in previous stories covering DNA damage-inducing agents. However, targeted therapy is able to selectively inhibit oncogenic proteins responsible for tumor progression. Imatinib (Gleevec) was the first compound used in targeted therapy to inhibit an oncogenic protein called BCR-ABL. BCR-ABL is a fusion protein encoded by the Philadelphia chromosome, which is generated by juxtaposing the ABL gene of chromosome 9 onto the BCR gene of chromosome 22. Dr. Peter Nowell from the University of Pennsylvania and David A. Hungerford from the Fox Chase Cancer Center together discovered the Philadelphia chromosome in 1959 and it after the city of the founding facilities.

BCR-ABL is a constitutively active tyrosine kinase that can upregulate several pro-survival pathways, making leukemia cells more aggressive and resistant to standard chemotherapies. As a result, BCR-ABL positive patients usually had high relapse rates and low survival rates prior to the discovery of Gleevec. Approximately 3%–5% of children and 25%–40% of adults diagnosed with acute lymphoblastic leukemia (ALL) have the BCR-ABL positive chromosome and poor prognosis. The survival rate of BCR-ABL positive pediatric patients was only 25% and was less than 20% for adult patients. Even worse, the BCR-ABL positive chromosome is present in more than 95% of chronic myeloid leukemia (CML) patients, which is also associated with poor diagnosis.

Fortunately, treatment options for ALL and CML was revolutionized when Gleevec was approved by the FDA in 2001. Clinical trials showed BCR-ABL-positive ALL patients who used Gleevec reached complete remission in more than 90% of patients with significantly lowered general toxicity as compared with general chemotherapy. For CML patients treated with Gleevec, the overall survival rate also increased to more than 80% as reported in a recent study. The discovery of Gleevec has caused a paradigm shift in treatment options for patients diagnosed with what was once seen as an almost incurable BC-ABL positive ALL and CML. However, resistance against Gleevec is starting to arise as seen in cancer cells that develop further mutations in the BCR-ABL gene. Second-generation BCR-ABL inhibitors including dasatinib, nilotinib, and bosutinib are being developed to be more potent than imatinib to overcome said resistance against Gleevec. In clinic practice, BCR-ABL inhibitors are often combined with traditional chemotherapy to treating BCR-ABL positive cancers.

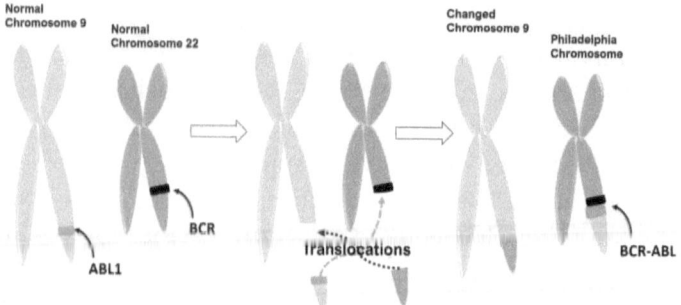

Figure 4.2: Translocation of DNA fragments between chromosome 9 and 22 generate a oncogenic protein called BCR-ABL. BCR-ABL is a kinase that can activate a myriad of downstream proteins that can promote cell survival.

Gleevec's success has paved a new way in prescribing tailored therapy based on which genetic mutations patients possess. Because drug targets are only present in malignant cells, the general toxicity is significantly lowered. As a result, Dr. Lyndon, who invented Gleevec, and Dr. Druker, who spearheaded the use of Gleevec in CML, were awarded with the Lasker-DeBakey Clinical Medical Research Award in 2009 for "converting a fatal cancer into a manageable condition."

There are still unanswered questions about the cause of BCR-ABL translocation and the risk factors that trigger the initiation of the translocation itself. If these risk factors were to be discovered, preventative measures can take place for individuals who are genetically predisposed to acquire the BCR-ABL translocation. Targeted therapy options for BCR-ABL negative leukemia patients are still limited, however. We will later discuss monoclonal antibodies, such as blinatumomab, that has brought new hope for BCR-ABL negative patients with relapsed or refractory ALL.

Reference

1. Nowell PC. Discovery of the Philadelphia chromosome: a personal perspective. J Clin Invest. 2007 Aug;117(8):2033-5.
2. Lugo TG, Pendergast AM, Muller AJ, Witte ON. Tyrosine kinase activity and transformation potency of bcr-abl oncogene products. Science. 1990 Mar 2;247(4946):1079-82.
3. Sánchez-García I, Grütz G. Tumorigenic activity of the BCR-ABL oncogenes is mediated by BCL2. Proc Natl Acad Sci U S A. 1995 Jun 6;92(12):5287-91.
4. Hochhaus A, Larson RA, Guilhot F, Radich JP,

Branford S, Hughes TP, Baccarani M, Deininger MW, Cervantes F, Fujihara S, Ortmann CE, Menssen HD, Kantarjian H, O'Brien SG, Druker BJ; IRIS Investigators. Long-Term Outcomes of Imatinib Treatment for Chronic Myeloid Leukemia. N Engl J Med. 2017 Mar 9;376(10):917-927.
5. Leoni V, Biondi A. Tyrosine kinase inhibitors in BCR-ABL positive acute lymphoblastic leukemia. Haematologica. 2015 Mar;100(3):295-9.
6. Skorski T. Genomic instability: The cause and effect of BCR/ABL tyrosine kinase. Curr Hematol Malig Rep. 2007 May;2(2):69-74.
7. Kantarjian H, Stein A, Gökbuget N, Fielding AK, Schuh AC, Ribera JM, Wei A, Dombret H, Foà R, Bassan R, Arslan Ö, Sanz MA, Bergeron J, Demirkan F, Lech-Maranda E, Rambaldi A, Thomas X, Horst HA, Brüggemann M, Klapper W, Wood BL, Fleishman A, Nagorsen D, Holland C, Zimmerman Z, Topp MS. Blinatumomab versus Chemotherapy for Advanced Acute Lymphoblastic Leukemia. N Engl J Med. 2017 Mar 2;376(9):836-847.

Epidermal growth factor receptor (EGFR) inhibitors - blocking signals by removing the antenna

Epidermal growth factor receptors (EGFRs) are located on cell membranes to receive and integrate extracellular signals to fine tune the growth and proliferation of tissue cells. Several genetically distinct ligands, including but not limited to EGF, transforming growth factor-α (TGF-α), and heparin-binding EGF, have been shown to bind to EGFR and activate signaling cascades. Perturbation of biofactor constitution in the extracellular compartment affects the activation status of EGFR, which disturbs distinct signaling pathways inside the cell. Given that changes in each downstream path of EGFR activation plays a vital role in tumorigenesis, we will only discuss the significance of EGFR in this section but will go into more detail of downstream pathways in subsequent stories.

A complete cascade of events is required to fully activate EGFRs. First, ligands must bind to EGFR to promote its dimerization, i.e., two parts of EGFR bind together to form a functional form of the receptor. Next, a part of the EGFR located inside the cell becomes phosphorylated, resulting in activation of the receptor itself. By understanding how EGFR is activated on a molecular level, we can fully appreciate the beauty in targeting specific activation steps for cancer therapy. For example, FDA-approved Nimotuzumab and Cetuximab are antibodies that work by specifically binding to EGFR, thus inhibiting binding of other EGFR ligands and keeping EGFR inactivated. Because malignant cells have high expression levels of EGFR, these antibodies ultimately block the progression of tumor cells.

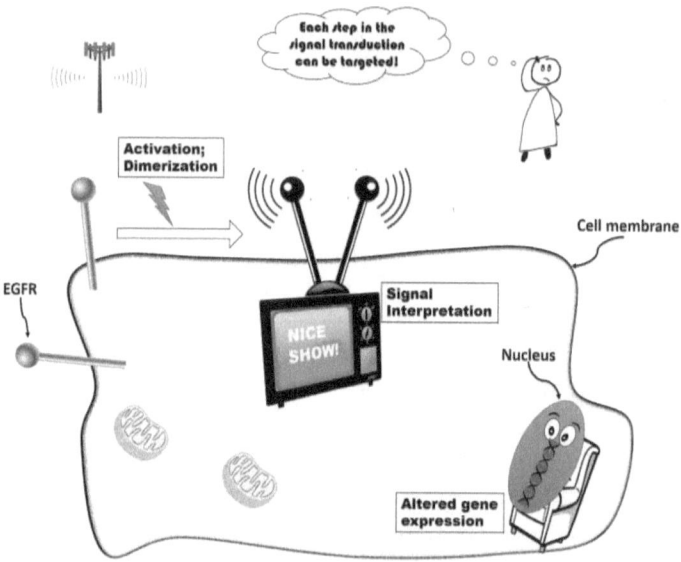

Figure 4.3: Uncontrolled activation of pro-survival EGFR signaling pathway will promote transcription of oncogenes that will promote tumorigenesis and progression.

As mentioned earlier, EGFR dimerization is one of the first steps of activating EGFR that is used as a target for cancer treatment. Antibody Pertuzumab was developed to block EGFR dimerization to prevent binding of EGFR ligands to inhibit triggering receptor activation. The FDA approved this novel compound in 2017 for the treatment of breast cancer. Just like EGFR ligand binding inhibitors, Pertuzumab keeps EGFR inactive to stop tumor progression.

Dimerization of EGFR also requires phosphorylation to become fully active, a process that is also targeted for specific inhibition of EGFR. Phosphorylation of EGFR is the final step required for EGFR activation that usually occurs spontaneously after dimerization through its active tyrosine kinase domain. Thus, tyrosine kinase inhibitors (TKIs) are used to keep EGFRs in its inactive/dephosphorylated form. This group of drugs include erlotinib, gefitinib and lapatinib, which are all widely used in practice for cancer treatment. However, cancer cells can overcome the effect of TKIs by inducing mutations in EGFR to weaken its inhibition. Fortunately, there are multiple TKIs available that physicians can prescribe for patients depending on their genetic alterations.

Use of EGFR inhibition for cancer treatment has made great strides in treating cancer. In addition, new TKIs are being developed that specifically target mutated forms of EGFR that oncologists can prescribe to tailor 'personalized' treatment regimens for their patients. In the following 5 sections, we will go over the EGFR-mediated downstream signaling pathways that are critical in tumor progression. A broad overview of how EGFR serves as an antenna that receives extracellular signals to act on certain downstream pathways will be summarized at the end of this section.

Reference
1. Berger C, Krengel U, Stang E, Moreno E, Madshus IH. Nimotuzumab and cetuximab block ligand-independent EGF receptor signaling efficiently at different concentrations. J Immunother. 2011 Sep;34(7):550-5.
2. Yang RY, Yang KS, Pike LJ, Marshall GR. Targeting the dimerization of epidermal growth factor receptors with small-molecule inhibitors. Chem Biol Drug Des. 2010 Jul;76(1):1-9.
3. Yewale C, Baradia D, Vhora I, Patil S, Misra A.

Epidermal growth factor receptor targeting in cancer: a review of trends and strategies. Biomaterials. 2013 Nov;34(34):8690-707.
4. Li S, Schmitz KR, Jeffrey PD, Wiltzius JJ, Kussie P, Ferguson KM. Structural basis for inhibition of the epidermal growth factor receptor by cetuximab. Cancer Cell. 2005 Apr;7(4):301-11.
5. Adams CW, Allison DE, Flagella K, Presta L, Clarke J, Dybdal N, McKeever K, Sliwkowski MX. Humanization of a recombinant monoclonal antibody to produce a therapeutic HER dimerization inhibitor, pertuzumab. Cancer Immunol Immunother. 2006 Jun;55(6):717-27.
6. Agus DB, Gordon MS, Taylor C, Natale RB, Karlan B, Mendelson DS, Press MF, Allison DE, Sliwkowski MX, Lieberman G, Kelsey SM, Fyfe G. Phase I clinical study of pertuzumab, a novel HER dimerization inhibitor, in patients with advanced cancer. J Clin Oncol. 2005 Apr 10;23(11):2534-43.
7. Morgillo F, Della Corte CM, Fasano M, Ciardiello F. Mechanisms of resistance to EGFR-targeted drugs: lung cancer. ESMO Open. 2016 May 11;1(3):e000060. eCollection 2016

Targeting MAPK pathway: too many mutations, not enough inhibitors

One of the pathways regulated by EGFR is the mitogen-activated protein kinase (MAPK) pathway that mediates the transduction of extracellular signals through intracellular signal transduction cascades. However, in malignant cells, components of this signaling cascade are often mutated, becoming hyper-activated and leading to uncontrolled cancer cell proliferation. It has been reported that approximately one-third of all cancers harbor genetic alterations that aberrantly upregulate MAPK-dependent signal transduction. The unchecked hyperactivation of the MAPK pathway has been shown as major momentum that drives tumorigeneses and progression in several types of human malignancies. Fortunately, scientists have developed inhibitors that downregulate this pathway by specifically targeting certain mutated forms of proteins within the cascade.

Mutated RAS proteins have been identified in colorectal, lung and pancreatic cancer. Up to 30% of all screened human cancers carry RAS mutations, making it a popular target for cancer treatment. However, RAS proteins are notorious for its lack of drug-binding sites, making it extremely difficult to develop effective RAS inhibitors. Instead, scientists have developed alternative ways to eradicate RAS activity by altering its post-translational modifications. Full activation of RAS proteins requires an association of RAS to the plasma membrane of a cell. Farnesylation, a post-translational attachment of lipid motifs, of RAS enables to become recruited to the cell membrane. Farnesyltransferase (FTase) inhibitors were developed to efficiently block the

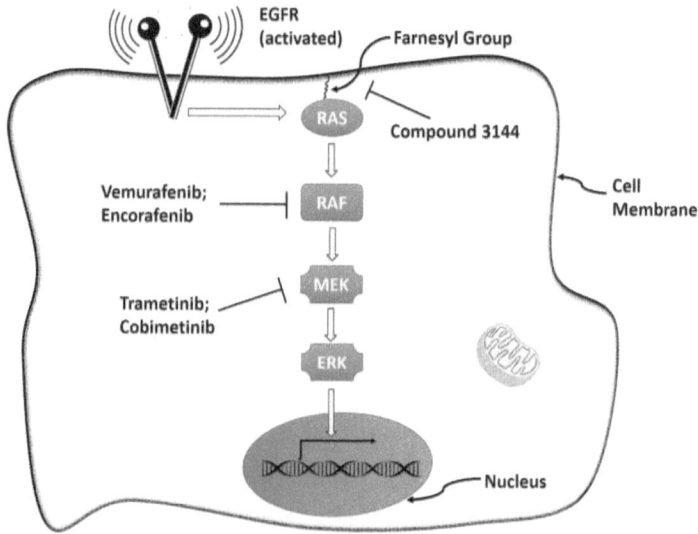

Figure 4.4: Compounds of the RAS/RAF/MEK/ERK signaling pathways have been identified mutated in many types of cancers. Targeted therapy against these mutated proteins has greatly improved the prognosis of cancer patients harboring these mutations.

membrane translocation of RAS. However, clinical trials of these compounds generally show limited efficacy. Fortunately, recent studies led by Dr. Stockwell using a new direct RAS inhibitor called compound 3144 has shown promising preclinical results.

Specific inhibitors of mutated forms of RAF protein, the downstream target of RAS, have been widely used in clinic for cancer treatment as well. An oncogenic mutation of a RAF protein called B-RAF is identified in 66% of malignant melanomas. Vemurafenib, one of the newer RAF inhibitors, has been clinically proven to be an efficient inhibitor of specific mutated forms of RAF in treating metastatic melanoma. Paradoxically, treatment of mutated RAF inhibitors can potentially induce dimerization of normal RAFs in healthy tissues cells. This can lead to hyperactivation of downstream MEK/ERK signaling and cell hyperproliferation, causing subcutaneous carcinoma and chronic lymphocytic leukemia (CLL) in a subset of patients treated with vemurafenib. A new generation of RAF inhibitors, such as Encorafenib, is currently undergoing multiple clinical trials to hopefully inhibit mutated RAF proteins without activating an oncogenic RAF-MEK-ERK cascade in wildtype tissue cells.

Targeting MEK1/2, major downstream compounds of the RAS/RAF signaling, has also been studied as a promising antitumor strategy. Mutations of MEK1/2 are often identified in relapsed/resistant cases because hyperactivation of MEK1/2 confers drug resistance by upregulating pro-survival proteins. In addition, tumors harboring MEK1/2 mutations are more likely to be resistant against inhibition of RAS and RAF proteins because ERK1/2 activation is highly dependent on MEK1/2 activation. In tumors harboring RAS and/or RAF mutations, inhibition of MEK1/2 can still render significant inhibition of ERK1/2, further highlighting the importance of developing MEK1/2 inhibitors. Thus, clinically approved MEK inhibitors Trametinib and Cobimetinib can be prescribed to cancer patients with cancer cells that have RAF mutations.

Reference

1. Uehling DE, Harris PA. Recent progress on MAP kinase pathway inhibitors. Bioorg Med Chem Lett. 2015 Oct 1;25(19):4047-56.
2. Martin GS. Cell signaling and cancer. Cancer Cell. 2003 Sep;4(3):167-74.
3. Forbes SA, Bindal N, Bamford S, Cole C, Kok CY, Beare D, Jia M, Shepherd R, Leung K, Menzies A, Teague JW, Campbell PJ, Stratton MR, Futreal PA. COSMIC: mining complete cancer genomes in the Catalogue of Somatic Mutations in Cancer. Nucleic Acids Res. 2011 Jan;39(Database issue):D945-50
4. Welsch ME, Kaplan A, Chambers JM, Stokes ME, Bos PH, Zask A, Zhang Y, Sanchez-Martin M, Badgley MA, Huang CS, Tran TH, Akkiraju H, Brown LM, Nandakumar R, Cremers S, Yang WS, Tong L, Olive KP, Ferrando A, Stockwell BR. Multivalent Small-Molecule Pan-RAS Inhibitors. Cell. 2017 Feb 23;168(5):878-889.e29.
5. Baines AT, Xu D, Der CJ. Inhibition of Ras for cancer treatment: the search continues. Future Med Chem. 2011 Oct;3(14):1787-808.
6. Yaktapour N, Meiss F, Mastroianni J, Zenz T, Andrlova H, Mathew NR, Claus R, Hutter B, Fröhling S, Brors B, Pfeifer D, Pantic M, Bartsch I, Spehl TS, Meyer PT, Duyster J, Zirlik K, Brummer T, Zeiser R. BRAF inhibitor-associated ERK activation drives development of chronic lymphocytic leukemia. J Clin Invest. 2014 Nov;124(11):5074-84.
7. Cheng Y, Tian H. Current Development Status of MEK Inhibitors. Molecules. 2017 Sep 26;22(10). pii: E1551

Mutations in PI3K pathway, how can we target you?

Extracellular signals are often needed for cells to upregulate protein synthesis level to get ready for proliferation and division when nutrients and growth factors are readily available. Growth factors bind to various cell membrane-localized receptors and activate downstream pathways. Upon growth factor binding, membrane-localized receptors mediate phosphoinositide 3-kinase (PI3K) activation which usually generates a second messenger called phosphatidylinositol-3,4,5-trisphosphate (PIP3). PIP3 in turn mediates activation of protein kinase B (AKT), which activates mTOR. PIP3, among other cellular chemicals, is usually called a second message, i.e., it can relay and amplify the initial signals (growth factors, in this case). A protein called PTEN inhibits this pathway by promoting de-phosphorylation of PIP3 to diminish the intensity of the signal. However, in malignant cells, tumor suppressor PTEN is mutated, rendering it dysfunctional.

The PI3K–AKT–mTOR pathway is one of the most critical pathways that increases protein synthesis. Activation of PI3K–AKT–mTOR signaling releases inhibitory mechanisms that maintain protein synthesis at low levels to allow cell growth and division. Mammalian Target of Rapamycin (mTOR) is a central control hub in mammalian cells that integrates various cellular stimuli to coordinate cell metabolism. Sufficient levels of oxygen, energy, amino acids, and growth factors all stimulate mTOR activation via the PI3K-AKT pathway.

Components of the PI3K–AKT–mTOR pathway are usually mutated or aberrantly activated in various cancers. Given the importance of mTOR hyperactivation in

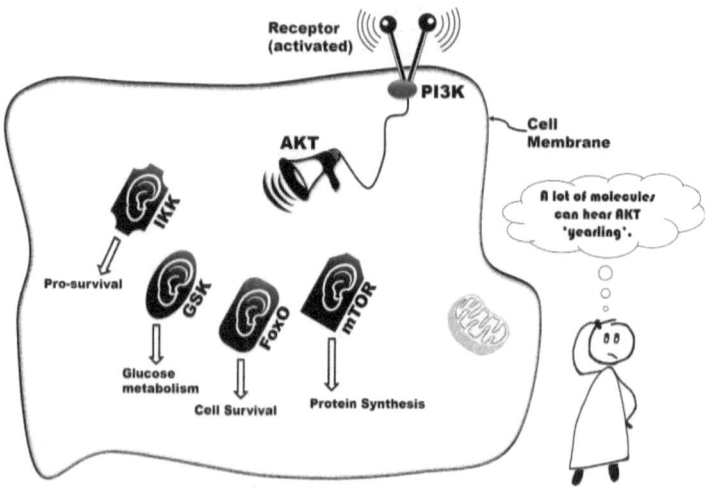

Figure 4.5: The PI3K/AKT signaling pathway has several downstream targets including IKK (NFkB pathway), GSK3, FOXO and mTOR. All these downstream targets play vital roles in promoting the survival of both normal and cancer cells.

mediating tumor progression, mTOR is specifically targeted during cancer treatment. The discovery for mTOR starts in early 1990s with the interesting finding that a bacteria-derived compound rapamycin or sirolimus was able to inhibit yeast growth. Shortly afterwards, in mid 1990s, mTOR was identified the target of rapamycin binding in mammalian cells and the PI3K-AKT-mTOR was later discovered as one of the main signaling cascade that regulates mTOR activation. Activation of mTOR will upregulate protein synthesis, cell cycle progression and promote cell survival. Since its discovery as an important mediator of cell growth and cell cycle progression, inhibition mTOR for cancer therapy was endeavored almost at the first day of its discovery. In 2007, the FDA approved Temsirolimus for use in treatment of advanced stage renal cell carcinoma, becoming the first mTOR inhibitor used in clinical practice for cancer treatment. Given the importance of mTOR in cell metabolism and energy regulation, there are inevitable side effects associated with long-term mTOR inhibitor use, including anemia, high blood sugar, and physical weakness.

Compared with the RAS-RAF-MEK-ERK signaling, the PI3K-AKT-mTOR pathway is more branched, meaning one upstream protein in its pathway usually has multiple downstream substrates. PI3K mutations are often associated with various types of cancers. In fact, in almost one out three cases of colorectal and colon cancer patients and one out of twelve cases for breast cancer patients were found to have PI3K mutations. Due to the existence of multiple PI3K isoforms and rising cases of resistance, developing PI3K inhibitors with clinical efficacy remains a daunting task for scientists. The first and yet only approved PI3K inhibitor used in cancer therapy is Buparlisib, which was approved by the FDA in 2014 for use against chronic lymphocytic leukemia (CLL).

Reference

1. Chalhoub N, Baker SJ. PTEN and the PI3-kinase pathway in cancer. Annu Rev Pathol. 2009;4:127-50.
2. Massacesi C, Di Tomaso E, Urban P, Germa C, Quadt C, Trandafir L, Aimone P, Fretault N, Dharan B, Tavorath R, Hirawat S. PI3K inhibitors as new cancer therapeutics: implications for clinical trial design. Onco Targets Ther. 2016 Jan 7;9:203-10.
3. Manning BD, Toker A. AKT/PKB Signaling: Navigating the Network. Cell. 2017 Apr 20;169(3):381-405.
4. Eng C. PTEN: one gene, many syndromes. Hum Mutat. 2003 Sep;22(3):183-98.
5. Samuels Y, Waldman T. Oncogenic mutations of PIK3CA in human cancers. Curr Top Microbiol Immunol. 2010;347:21-41. doi: 10.1007/82_2010_68.
6. Massacesi C, Di Tomaso E, Urban P, Germa C, Quadt C, Trandafir L, Aimone P, Fretault N, Dharan B, Tavorath R, Hirawat S. PI3K inhibitors as new cancer therapeutics: implications for clinical trial design. Onco Targets Ther. 2016 Jan 7;9:203-10.
7. Bellmunt J, Szczylik C, Feingold J, Strahs A, Berkenblit A. Temsirolimus safety profile and management of toxic effects in patients with advanced renal cell carcinoma and poor prognostic features. Ann Oncol. 2008 Aug;19(8):1387-92.

Bcl-2 inhibition, tipping the balance towards cell death

A key concept in understanding cell survival at a molecular level is to keep the levels of pro and anti-survival proteins balanced. In mammalian cells, this balance is mediated by a group of proteins called B cell CLL/lymphoma-2 (BCL-2) family proteins. Pro-death BCL-2 proteins, including Bax, Bak, BID, BIM and NOXA, are responsible for inducing formation of pores on the membranes of mitochondria. This leads to the release of cytochrome c into the cytoplasm, which triggers a cascade of events eventually kills the cell. Essentially, the membrane of the "powerhouse" of a cell acts as a dam, within which contains energy to sustain a community. These pro-death factors infiltrate the dam, leading to a massive breach that floods the community. Bax and Bak proteins are evenly distributed in the mitochondrial membrane to maintain its structural integrity. Activated BIM and NOXA interact with Bax and Bak to cause clustering of Bax and Bak proteins, which leads to the formation of pores in the mitochondria membrane to cause depolarization of the cell.

Since activation of pro-death BCL-2 family proteins is almost the final step that can lead to activation of self-destruction, a delicate regulatory mechanism is involved to strictly regulate this process. A group of pro-survival BCL-2 family protein including Bcl-2, Mcl-1, Puma and Bcl-xL specifically functions to bind those pro-death BCL-2 family proteins to keep them in inactivated form. As we all know, resistance to death is one of the hallmarks of cancer cells. To achieve that by deactivating

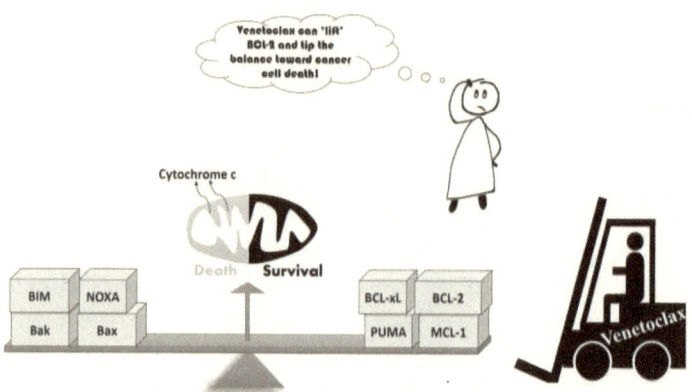

Figure 4.6: The balance between pro-survival (BCL-xL, BCL-2, PUMA, MCL-2, etc.) and apoptotic (BIM, NOXA, Bak, Bax, etc.) proteins are required for cell survival. Inhibition of the pro-survival Bcl-2 protein using its specific inhibitor Venetoclax can tip the balance towards cell death.

pro-death proteins either via downregulating transcription of pro-death proteins or upregulating pro-survival BCL-2 family proteins. It is possible for cancer cells to have higher cellular levels of pro-survival BCL-2 family proteins in order to escape death or to develop resistance against anti-tumor therapies. Thus, Bax and Bak proteins in cancer cells are usually kept in their inactive form, rendering chemotherapy impotent in inducing cancer cell death.

To promote cell survival, the amount of pro-survival BCL-2 family proteins and pro-death proteins need to be balanced to prevent Bax and Bak clustering in the mitochondrial membrane. In cancer therapy, we want to interrupt this balance so that pro-death proteins overwhelm pro-survival proteins to promote cancer cell death. As simple as this sounds, scientists have worked on this idea for several decades to develop such a compound that can hijack this balance.

Currently, the most successful strategy that disturbs this balance works through specific inhibition of BCL-2 to prevent its pro-survival effects. In 2016, the first BCL-2 inhibitor, venetoclax, was approved by the FDA for use in treatment of high-risk relapsed chronic lymphocytic leukemia (CLL). CLL cells express unusually high levels of BCL-2 proteins as one of its major oncogenic features. Use of venetoclax inactivates the pro-survival BCL-2 protein to tip the balance in favor of cell death, making them susceptible to other forms of cancer therapy. This is one major reason why in multiple ongoing clinical trials, venetoclax is usually combined with other chemotherapeutic agents. However, in other types of cancer, cell survival is not as dependent on BCL-2. Instead, they are more dependent on upregulated Mcl-1 and/or Bxl-xL for survival and resistance.

The pro and anti-survival groups of BCL-2 family proteins need to be balanced like Yin and Yang to promote survival and body wellness. Diseases in general occur due to imbalance of this Yin and Yang within cells.

Shuhua (Steve) Zheng, Ph.D.

Reference
1. Cang S, Iragavarapu C, Savooji J, Song Y, Liu D. ABT-199 (venetoclax) and BCL-2 inhibitors in clinical development. J Hematol Oncol. 2015 Nov 20;8:129.
2. Rossé T, Olivier R, Monney L, Rager M, Conus S, Fellay I, Jansen B, Borner C. Bcl-2 prolongs cell survival after Bax-induced release of cytochrome c. Send to Nature. 1998 Jan 29;391(6666):496-9.
3. Murphy KM, Streips UN, Lock RB. Bax membrane insertion during Fas(CD95)-induced apoptosis precedes cytochrome c release and is inhibited by Bcl-2. Send to Oncogene. 1999 Oct 28;18(44):5991-9.
4. Chipuk JE, Moldoveanu T, Llambi F, Parsons MJ, Green DR. The BCL-2 family reunion. Mol Cell. 2010 Feb 12;37(3):299-310.
5. Anderson MA, Deng J, Seymour JF, Tam C, Kim SY, Fein J, Yu L, Brown JR, Westerman D, Si EG, Majewski IJ, Segal D, Heitner Enschede SL, Huang DC, Davids MS, Letai A, Roberts AW. The BCL2 selective inhibitor venetoclax induces rapid onset apoptosis of CLL cells in patients via a TP53-independent mechanism. Blood. 2016 Jun 23;127(25):3215-24.
6. Cang S, Iragavarapu C, Savooji J, Song Y, Liu D. ABT-199 (venetoclax) and BCL-2 inhibitors in clinical development. J Hematol Oncol. 2015 Nov 20;8:129.

Shuhua (Steve) Zheng, Ph.D.

CHAPTER V: IMMUNOTHERAPY

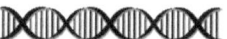

"Though the idea of using the immune system to fight neoplastic disease was novel in the 1980s, its practice was not. William B. Coley, a nineteenth century surgeon at the Hospital for the Ruptured and Crippled (now the Hospital for Special Surgery), developed the first immune-based treatment for cancer at the end of the nineteenth century."

William K. Decker, Ph.D.

" Nature often gives us hints to her profoundest secrets, and it is possible that she has given us a hint which, if we will but follow, may lead us to on to the solution of this difficult problem (sarcoma). "

William B. Coley, M.D.

"Anti-CTLA4 therapy strongly enhances the amplitude of vaccine-induced antitumor responses in many poorly immunogenic tumor models, as does anti-PD1 therapy."

Drew M. Pardoll, M.D., Ph.D.

Introduction

New discoveries in cancer immunotherapy are often headliners worldwide showcasing several new drugs approved by the FDA to bring new hopes for the treatment of even the deadliest types of human malignancies. The use of immunotherapy to treat cancer dates as far back to the 1890s when Dr. William B. Coley, who at the time was in his late 20s, was the first physician who systematically studied and practiced immunotherapy for his cancer patients. In his practice, Dr. Coley injected over a thousand of his cancer patients with bacteria or bacterial products (later known as Coley's Toxins). He and other physicians who also performed bacterial injections, reported excellent results, especially in cases that involved bone and soft-tissue sarcomas. However, due to lack of understanding of the mechanism of action behind his treatment strategy, coupled with subsequent advent of chemotherapy and radiation therapy, use of Coley's Toxins gradually disappeared from the realm of medicine. But because Dr. Coley's toxins had benefitted many cancer patients during a period when very little was known about how the immune system functioned, experts today credit him as the "Father of Immunotherapy" for his pioneering work.

So, what is immunotherapy and why did the founding father of immunotherapy use potentially harmful bacterial to fight cancer? Before we explain this, we must first understand that cancer cells originate from normal cells but have the added ability to evade immune surveillance. Luckily, an uncompromised immune system can usually detect abnormal cells with cancerous mutations. However, some cancer cells have evolved to gain mechanisms that allow them to hide their abnormalities, allowing unchecked continuous growth. Injecting detrimental bacterial near tumors causes local accumulation of immune cells to fight the bacterial infection. It is possible that those the local accumulation of immune cells can additionally target nearby tumors. However, it is important to note that deleterious side effects can occur with this methodology due to the lack of specificity and inherent unpredictability.

Although "first-generation" immunotherapy methods were crude, modern immunotherapies are tailored to specifically target "non-self" markers expressed by tumor cells. In the human body, a group of immune cells called cytotoxic T cells (a.k.a., CD8+ T-cells) are mainly responsible for recognizing and eradicating tumor cells. These T-cells are the major guardians against intracellular pathogens that infect host tissue cells. For examples, for tissue cells infected with virus, the viral genome will be incorporated in the host cells and sometimes become part of host cells' genome. By doing that, the virus will be capable of hibernating and hiding away from host's immune system. However, when the virus starts to replicate and produce viral proteins, some of those proteins will be processed into peptides (small fragments of proteins) and presented to the host cell surface by the major histocompatibility complex (MHC). The viral peptides presented will be readily recognized by T cells which will then develop into a group of T cells carrying a receptor specific for that MHC-viral peptide complex. Those cytotoxic T cells will kill the cells presenting viral peptide and thus preventing the expansion of virus in the host. The physical interaction between MHC-peptide complex and T cell receptor that recognizes the complex is critical in successful activation of cytotoxic T cells. Either too strong or too weak of the binding will make the T cell energic and unable to elicit efficient killing. However, to prevent cytotoxic T-cells from mistakenly targeting healthy tissue cells and cause autoimmune diseases, our body system has developed several "checkpoints" that T-cells must pass in order to develop into fully functional cytotoxic T cells.

During tumor growth in immunocompetent individuals, some T-cells indeed have developed antitumor specificity since some tumor cells also present unusual MHC-peptide complexes that T cells recognize as non-self antigens. However, tumor cells often evade destruction by suppressing proliferation of these cytotoxic T-cells so that they cannot reach an effective population size. To combat this, scientists have developed strategies to override suppression and promote clonal proliferation of antitumor T-cells so that they can help eradicate the tumor. The most straightforward method is to isolate tumor-targeting T-cells from a patient's biopsies, culture them in-vitro, and inject the populated T-cells back into the patient. Unfortunately, it is difficult to precisely obtain solely the T-cells that are specific in targeting tumor cells. Thus, another method has been developed to work around this obstacle known as chimeric antigen receptor (CAR) T-cell therapy. CAR therapy involves directly editing a patient's genome to create a gene that encodes for tumor-specific receptors to be inserted directly into onto T-cells. By doing so, scientists and physicians can basically create a very specific antitumor T cells populations that specifically designed for that patient. This groundbreaking technology will create a living 'drug' that is derived from the patient and then specifically designed to kill the tumor cells in that patient.

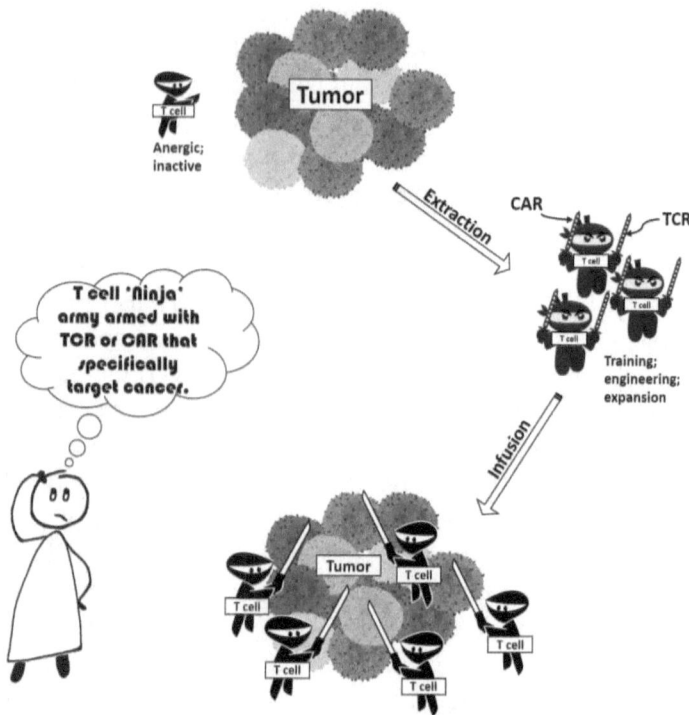

Figure 5.1: Cytotoxic T can be extracted from cancer patients either from circulation or biopsy of tumor masses. The derived T cells can be engineered to express receptors express tumor specific receptors. Some tumor infiltrating T-lymphocytes (TILs) already have anti-tumor specificity. They can be populated in the lab and infused back into the patient for therapeutic gain.

Other strategies that show promising clinical trial results involve direct stimulation of cytotoxic T-cell growth in cancer patients by inhibiting checkpoints that downregulate T-cell development. As discussed previously, hyperactivation of cytotoxic T-cells are potentially detrimental as it may lead to autoimmune diseases. Another pitfall to this strategy is that all forms of cytotoxic T-cells are 'stimulated' to attack their targets, which can lead to further detrimental side effects.

Immunotherapy is not only successful in treating cancer but also in preventing cancer formation. This explains why that compared with immuno-competent people, immunosuppressed patients (patients with HIV infection, transplants, etc.) are more susceptible to have cancer and worse prognosis once diagnosed. As you may know, extrapolating the concept of creating vaccines to prevent infectious diseases, one may ask, can we also develop vaccines against malignancies? To do so, scientists need to ascertain the leading cause of specific types of tumors. For example, human papillomavirus (HPV) is a major cause of cervical cancer and oropharyngeal cancers. Consequently, HPV vaccines decrease the risk of acquiring HPV infections, thus protecting us from cervical and oropharyngeal cancers. Although promising, cancers that are not of viral origin prove difficult for scientists to develop anti-cancer vaccines.

Another branch of the immune system that has the potential to trigger anti-tumor effects is humoral immunity. In humoral immunity, B-cells produce antibodies that can bind to tumors to label them for destruction. In addition, B-cells can also release cytotoxic cytokines that facilitate the anti-tumor effects of T-cells. At this time, scientists only have an elementary understanding of how B-cells are implicated in tumorigenesis and progression. This chapter will focus on cutting-edge technologies that engineer T-cells to become cancer-killing machines.

Reference
1. Coley WB. The treatment of malignant tumors by repeated inoculations of erysipelas. With a report of ten original cases. 1893. Clin Orthop Relat Res. 1991 Jan;(262):3-11.
2. McCarthy EF. The toxins of William B. Coley and the treatment of bone and soft-tissue sarcomas. Iowa Orthop J. 2006;26:154-8.
3. Miliotou AN, Papadopoulou LC. CAR T-cell Therapy: A New Era in Cancer Immunotherapy. Curr Pharm Biotechnol. 2018;19(1):5-18.
4. Koch U, Radtke F. Mechanisms of T cell development and transformation. Annu Rev Cell Dev Biol. 2011;27:539-62.
5. Montagna D, Schiavo R, Gibelli N, Pedrazzoli P, Tonelli R, Pagani S, Assirelli E, Locatelli F, Pession A, Fregoni V, Montini E, Da Prada GA, Siena S, Maccario R. Ex vivo generation and expansion of anti-tumor cytotoxic T-cell lines derived from patients or their HLA-identical sibling. Int J Cancer. 2004 May 20;110(1):76-86.
6. Farkona S, Diamandis EP, Blasutig IM. Cancer immunotherapy: the beginning of the end of cancer? BMC Med. 2016 May 5;14:73.
7. Yee C, Thompson JA, Byrd D, Riddell SR, Roche P, Celis E, Greenberg PD. Adoptive T cell therapy using antigen-specific CD8+ T cell clones for the treatment of patients with metastatic melanoma: in vivo persistence, migration, and antitumor effect of

transferred T cells. Proc Natl Acad Sci U S A. 2002 Dec 10;99(25):16168-73.
8. Bu X, Yao Y, Li X. Immune Checkpoint Blockade in Breast Cancer Therapy. Adv Exp Med Biol. 2017;1026:383-402.
9. Silverberg MJ, Chao C, Leyden WA, Xu L, Horberg MA, Klein D, Towner WJ, Dubrow R, Quesenberry CP Jr, Neugebauer RS, Abrams DI. HIV infection, immunodeficiency, viral replication, and the risk of cancer. Cancer Epidemiol Biomarkers Prev. 2011 Dec;20(12):2551-9.
10. Roden RBS, Stern PL. Opportunities and challenges for human papillomavirus vaccination in cancer. Nat Rev Cancer. 2018 Apr;18(4):240-254.
11. Doorbar J, Egawa N, Griffin H, Kranjec C, Murakami I. Human papillomavirus molecular biology and disease association. Rev Med Virol. 2015 Mar;25 Suppl 1:2-23.
12. Yuen GJ, Demissie E, Pillai S. B lymphocytes and cancer: a love-hate relationship. Trends Cancer. 2016 Dec;2(12):747-757.

Shuhua (Steve) Zheng, Ph.D.

Adoptive T-cell therapy – Reviving tumor infiltrating T-lymphocytes (TILs)

Tumor cells usually bear genetic mutations that are largely responsible for the development of malignant features such as uncontrolled cell growth, loss of cell-cell contact and poor differentiation. These mutations often alter peptide-MHC (pMHC) complexes that are present on the surface of cancer cells. If these complexes are recognized by T-cells, it leads to to development of tumor-specific T-cells. Tumor-recognizing T-cells are called tumor infiltrating T lymphocytes (TILs) and can be isolated from tumor biopsies for further study and expansion. In many cases, tumor cells evade the surveillance of TILs by either secreting cytokines that dampen TIL functionality or by upregulating local presence a specific group of cells called regulatory T cells (Treg) to suppress anti-tumor immune responses. In tumors that are caused by viruses, the MHC protein expression is inhibited so that not as much tumor-specific pMHC are presented. By doing so, tumor cells can evade immune surveillance and develop uncontrolled growth. So how can we upregulate anti-tumor effects of TILs?

The anti-tumor effects of TILs were first identified and depicted back in 1980s led by Dr. Rosenberg's team. The TILs in their study were deprived from tumor biopsies of 6 patients with metastatic melanoma and interestingly, more than 30 years after that initial study, clinical trials on TILs still aims metastatic melanoma for potential therapeutic improvement of this horrible disease. So why scientists believe melanoma can be efficiently targeted by TILs? While other types of malignancies may have different mechanisms for tumor

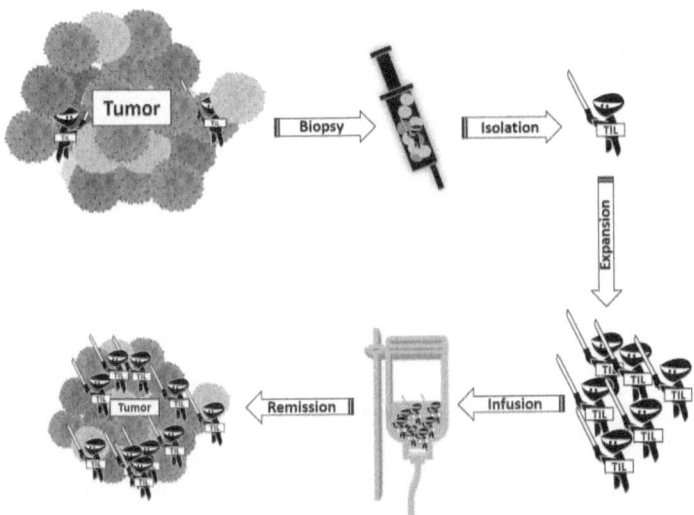

Figure 5.2: Tumor infiltrating T-lymphocytes have anti-tumor activity. They are isolated from the biopsy of the tumor mass and repopulated in vitro. Then, they will be infused back into the patient to kill cancer cells.

development, the initiation and progression of melanoma in populations of European origin are well proven associated accumulation of genetic mutations from sunburn. As a result, melanoma cells are highly likely to carry multiple altered proteins that will be processed and recognized by TILs. Also, with accumulation of genetic mutations, those melanoma cells are more likely to develop resistance to traditional chemotherapies, further highlighting the importance of TIL-mediated immunotherapy for malignant melanoma.

The ultimate goal in TIL-mediated immunotherapy is to improve the presence of tumor-specific TIL in the tumor mass to overwhelm the immuno-suppressive mechanisms deployed by tumor cells. TIL-mediated immunotherapy begins with taking a tumor biopsy. TILs are then isolated from the biopsy sample and expanded in-vitro. Upon reaching a suitable population size of TILs, physicians will infuse them into the patient together will the cytokine Interleukin 2 (IL-2) to help maintain T-cell viability. Afterwards, the physician regularly monitors the tumor to evaluate therapeutic efficacy. In some cases, radiation and chemotherapies will used as supplemental therapy to target the patient's bone marrow to decrease the amount of Treg cells, which among other cells that can inhibit the efficacy of the reinfused TILs. TILs originate from the patient him/herself, this treatment strategy is called adoptive T cell therapy (ACT), which has gone through multiple clinical trials in the last decade, confirming its safety. TIL-mediated ACT is especially useful in fighting cancer cells that have developed resistance to traditional pharmaceutical strategies. Because multiple antigens are present on the surface of tumor cells, TILs can target a cohort of tumor-specific antigens making cancer cells susceptible to TIL-mediated ACT.

Since traditional chemo-/radio-therapies will, to some degree, suppress immune responses due to off-target side effects, will they dampen the efficacy of TILs? Studies have shown that chemo;/radio-therapy causes cancer cell lysis, which releases their content directly into the body's extracellular compartment. If non-self proteins are present, this actually helps the immune system develop an anti-tumor response. Indeed, multiple undergoing Phase II clinical trials are combining chemo-/radio-therapies with TIL-mediated immunotherapy for better clinical outcomes. However, the inherent barriers to widespread clinical application of TIL-mediated immunotherapy is the cost due to complicated processes involved in isolation and expansion of tumor-specific TILs. Thus, only few patients can afford this treatment because most insurance companies may deny coverage for TIL-mediated cell therapy. More efforts are definitely needed to lower the costs associated with the treatment to benefit more cancer patients.

Reference
1. Muul LM, Spiess PJ, Director EP, Rosenberg SA. Identification of specific cytolytic immune responses against autologous tumor in humans bearing malignant melanoma. J Immunol. 1987 Feb 1;138(3):989-95.
2. Newton-Bishop JA, Chang YM, Elliott F, Chan M, Leake S, Karpavicius B, Haynes S, Fitzgibbon E, Kukalizch K, Randerson-Moor J, Elder DE, Bishop DT, Barrett JH. Relationship between sun exposure and melanoma risk for tumours in different body sites in a large case-control study in a temperate climate. Eur J Cancer. 2011 Mar;47(5):732-41.
3. Wu S, Singh RK. Resistance to chemotherapy and molecularly targeted therapies: rationale for combination therapy in malignant melanoma. Curr Mol Med. 2011 Oct;11(7):553-63.
4. Cruz CR, Hanley PJ, Liu H, Torrano V, Lin YF, Arce JA, Gottschalk S, Savoldo B, Dotti G, Louis CU, Leen AM, Gee AP, Rooney CM, Brenner MK, Bollard CM, Heslop HE. Adverse events following infusion of T cells for adoptive immunotherapy: a 10-year experience. Cytotherapy. 2010 Oct;12(6):743-9.
5. Rosenberg SA, Yang JC, Sherry RM, Kammula US, Hughes MS, Phan GQ, Citrin DE, Restifo NP, Robbins PF, Wunderlich JR, Morton KE, Laurencot CM, Steinberg SM, White DE, Dudley ME. Durable complete responses in heavily pretreated patients with

metastatic melanoma using T-cell transfer immunotherapy.
6. Wu R, Forget MA, Chacon J, Bernatchez C, Haymaker C, Chen JQ, Hwu P, Radvanyi LG. Adoptive T-cell therapy using autologous tumor-infiltrating lymphocytes for metastatic melanoma: current status and future outlook. Cancer J. 2012 Mar-Apr;18(2):160-75.

Finding a needle in a haystack – T-cell receptor-engineered T-cell therapy

While TIL-based adoptive T-cell therapy have brought new hopes for patients with melanoma, for patients with other caners, isolating and expanding pre-existing tumor-reacting T-cells still proves to be a daunting task. To overcome this, scientists have developed new strategies by directly 'inserting' tumor-recognizing T-cell receptors (TCRs) into patients to directly attach to their T-cells. The TCR is a receptor complex that is expressed on T-cells that recognize peptide major histocompatibility complex (pMHC). The binding between TCR and pMHC is a prerequisite for T-cell mediated cell death of targeted cells. Ideally, the inserted TCR guides T-cells to hunt for tumor cells that express the corresponding pMHC. In TCR-engineered T-cell therapy, we can 'instruct' cytotoxic T-cells to go after specific tumor cells expressing mutated pMHC. By doing so, TCR therapy can theoretically be engineered to target any type of cancer.

However, the steps involved in the generation of TCR-engineered T-cells that specifically target cancer cells are quite challenging due to complicated biomedical engineering techniques needed. The first step involves identifying tumor-specific antigens that are targeted by the TCR. Next, a tumor biopsy is performed to sequence the genome of its cells to look for specific mutations. Protein peptides corresponding to mutated DNA sequences were synthesized and used to stimulate naive T-cells to generate corresponding TCRs. DNA sequence corresponding to that specific TCR are sequenced is then engineered into vectors. Those vectors carrying the gene

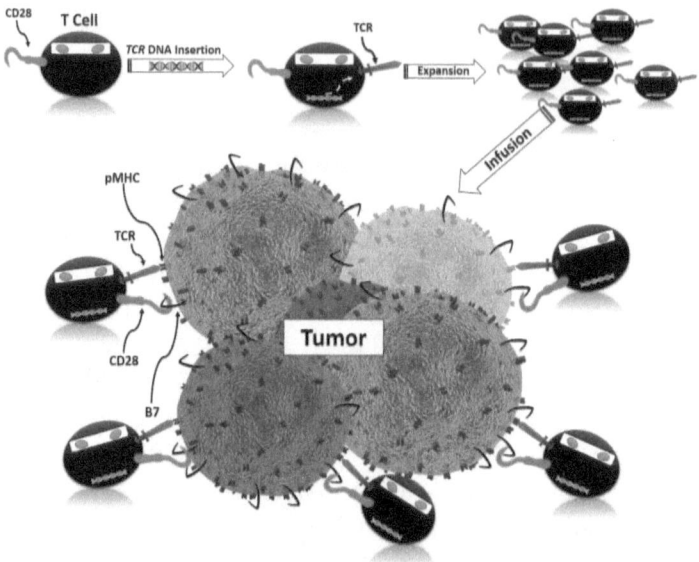

Figure 5.3: Cytotoxic T cells derived from the patient can be armed with tumor specific T cell receptors (TCRs). The TCR together with the costimulatory receptor CD28 can work together to specifically eradicate cancer cells.

encoding tumor-specific TCR will insert into the genome of the T cells derived from the patient. At the end, the T cells in the patients are now armed with TCRs that can recognize tumor specific antigens. Clinical trials using TCR-engineered T-cell therapy has shown success in treating colorectal carcinoma, metastatic melanoma, synovial sarcoma, and multiple myeloma.

However, using engineered T-cells have an inherent risk of developing cross-reactivity against normal tissue cells. For example, T-cells that are engineered to target melanoma cells can also target melanocytic cells present in the skin, eyes and inner ears, causing damages to normal tissue cells. Other side effects include severe cardiac toxicity possible due to unexpected cross reactivity with proteins that exist in the cardiac muscle. These side effects are amplified by the fact that every person has their own unique immune system with different sensitivities and immune regulatory mechanisms. To avoid those shortcomings, scientists are researching new antigens that allow for better specificity without cross-reactivity.

Another inherent shortcoming with TCR-engineered T-cell therapy is that T-cells already carry TCRs for non-tumor antigens. Thus, there are potential adverse effects with infusing a large population of cytotoxic T cells that carry two sets of TCRs, one against tumor and one against an unknown antigen. Fortunately, scientists have developed strategies to downregulate the expression of the initial set of TCRs to allow almost only the tumor-specific TCRs to be expressed prior to infusion. TCR-engineered T-cell therapy is now under Phase I/II clinical trials against both hematological malignancies and solid tumors.

Reference

1. Ping Y, Liu C, Zhang Y. T-cell receptor-engineered T cells for cancer treatment: current status and future directions. Protein Cell. 2018 Mar;9(3):254-266.
2. Ikeda H. T-cell adoptive immunotherapy using tumor-infiltrating T cells and genetically engineered TCR-T cells. Int Immunol. 2016 Jul;28(7):349-53.
3. Matsuda T, Leisegang M, Park JH, Ren L, Kato T, Ikeda Y, Harada M, Kiyotani K, Lengyel E, Fleming

GF, Nakamura Y. Induction of Neoantigen-specific Cytotoxic T Cells and Construction of T-cell Receptor-engineered T cells for Ovarian Cancer. Clin Cancer Res. 2018 May 2. pii: clincanres.0142.2018.
4. Lu YC, Zheng Z, Robbins PF, Tran E, Prickett TD, Gartner JJ, Li YF, Ray S, Franco Z, Bliskovsky V, Fitzgerald PC, Rosenberg SA. An Efficient Single-Cell RNA-Seq Approach to Identify Neoantigen-Specific T Cell Receptors. Mol Ther. 2018 Feb 7;26(2):379-389.
5. Robbins PF, Kassim SH, Tran TL, Crystal JS, Morgan RA, Feldman SA, Yang JC, Dudley ME, Wunderlich JR, Sherry RM, Kammula US, Hughes MS, Restifo NP, Raffeld M, Lee CC, Li YF, El-Gamil M, Rosenberg SA. A pilot trial using lymphocytes genetically engineered with an NY-ESO-1-reactive T-cell receptor: long-term follow-up and correlates with response. Clin Cancer Res. 2015 Mar 1;21(5):1019-27.
6. Linette GP, Stadtmauer EA, Maus MV, Rapoport AP, Levine BL, Emery L, Litzky L, Bagg A, Carreno BM, Cimino PJ, Binder-Scholl GK, Smethurst DP, Gerry AB, Pumphrey NJ, Bennett AD, Brewer JE, Dukes J, Harper J, Tayton-Martin HK, Jakobsen BK, Hassan NJ, Kalos M, June CH. Cardiovascular toxicity and titin cross-reactivity of affinity-enhanced T cells in myeloma and melanoma. Blood. 2013 Aug 8;122(6):863-71.
7. Provasi E, Genovese P, Lombardo A, Magnani Z, Liu PQ, Reik A, Chu V, Paschon DE, Zhang L, Kuball J, Camisa B, Bondanza A, Casorati G, Ponzoni M, Ciceri F, Bordignon C, Greenberg PD, Holmes MC, Gregory PD, Naldini L, Bonini C. Editing T cell specificity towards leukemia by zinc finger nucleases and lentiviral gene transfer. Nat Med. 2012 May;18(5):807-815.

CAR T-cell therapy, a promise for cancer cure?

While TIL and TCR-engineered T-cell therapies have paved new avenues in cancer treatment, both have inherent shortcomings associated with limited applicability and technological complexities, respectively. We want to have a T-cell therapy that can be applied to several types of cancer at a relatively affordable price. Recent development in chimeric antigen receptor (CAR) T-cell therapy may find the key to this problem. Before we discuss what CAR T-cell therapy is and why it is unique, we must first understand the steps involved in activating T-cells from a naïve cell.

T-cells are first developed in the thymus and migrate to lymph nodes in which its TCRs interact with peptide major histocompatibility complex (pMHC) present on antigen presenting cells (APCs). Then, a second costimulatory signal, the interaction between CD28 and B7 molecules presented on T-cells and APCs, respectively, is triggered. This costimulatory signal activates several downstream pathways that cause cytokine production, such as interleukin-2 (IL-2) which is required for full activation and proliferation of T-cells. Without IL-2, T cells become anergic and undergo apoptosis. This delicate system helps prompt activation of the immune system when non-self antigens are presented by APCs.

If we want to turn T-cells into cancer killer cells, we also need to provide these two signals for T-cells that are already activated with anti-tumor TCRs. You can also reinvent the wheel by integrating these two signals into one single receptor in T cells. Scientists have implemented this idea by creating a brand-new antigen

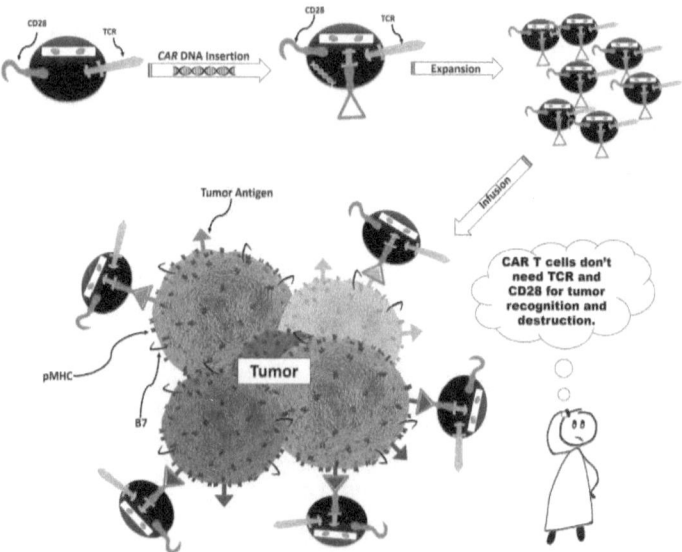

Figure 5.4: T cell derived from the cancer patient can be engineered to express chimeric antigen receptor (CAR) that have tumor specificity. Binding between CAR and tumor specific antigens will activate the CAR-T cells to kill cancer cells. The costimulatory receptor CD 28 is not required for CAR-T cell activation.

receptor called the chimeric antigen receptor (CAR) that can specifically bind antigen and upon doing that, directly activate the intracellular part of CAR and trigger strong downstream activation signal that will also leads to IL-2 transcription. Thus, T cells with CARs can be activated independent from MHC and the CD28-mediated costimulatory signal. The CAR was constructed in a similar fashion as LEGO creations. An antibody with anti-tumor specificity is 'connected' with structural 'bricks' derived from intracellular parts of CD3 and CD28, which are responsible for relaying signals upon

TCR and costimulation activation, respectively. Thus, binding of CAR to antigens present on tumor cells simultaneously activates the required 1st and co-stimulatory signals, leading to the development of T-cells with anti-tumor activities. The CAR basically made a short-cut so that T cells can be empowered with anti-tumor activity without having to go through complicated activation steps developed by Mother Nature. Because DNA is easily 'editable' with modern biotechniques, we are capable of developing any CAR T-cell for new tumor antigens identified in any cancers. For tumor cells that express low levels of targetable antigens, T-cells can be engineered to express higher levels of CAR to increase selectivity for these tumor cells. For tumors expressing more than one targetable antigen, T-cells can be inserted with two sets of CARs to target their separate antigens.

All these unique features have made CAR a popular research topic within the last 25 years. In 2017, the FDA approved CAR T-cell therapy for the treatment of acute lymphoblastic leukemia. The antigen targeted by CAR T-cell in ALL is CD19, which is prevalent and highly expressed in B-cell malignancies. However, clinical trials have shown that around 28% of pediatric and young adult patients with acute leukemia develop resistance to CAR T-cell therapy via downregulation of CD19, rendering CAR T-cells unable to find their target. Also, infusion of a large amount of T-cells can potentially cause cytokine release syndrome, a severe side effect that requires immediate medical attention. Despite these setbacks, new targetable antigens are constantly being discovered and several clinical trials are currently in place to evaluate the efficacy of CAR T-cell therapy in treating many types of cancer.

Reference

1. Koch U, Radtke F. Mechanisms of T cell development and transformation. Annu Rev Cell Dev Biol. 2011;27:539-62.
2. Hartmann J, Schüßler-Lenz M, Bondanza A4, Buchholz CJ. Clinical development of CAR T cells-challenges and opportunities in translating innovative treatment concepts. EMBO Mol Med. 2017 Sep;9(9):1183-1197.
3. June CH, O'Connor RS, Kawalekar OU, Ghassemi S, Milone MC. CAR T cell immunotherapy for human cancer. Science. 2018 Mar 23;359(6382):1361-1365.
4. van Zelm MC, Reisli I, van der Burg M, Castaño D, van Noesel CJ, van Tol MJ, Woellner C, Grimbacher B, Patiño PJ, van Dongen JJ, Franco JL. An antibody-deficiency syndrome due to mutations in the CD19 gene. N Engl J Med. 2006 May 4;354(18):1901-12.
5. Dotti G, Gottschalk S, Savoldo B, Brenner MK. Design and development of therapies using chimeric antigen receptor-expressing T cells. Immunol Rev. 2014 Jan;257(1):107-26.
6. Maude SL, Laetsch TW, Buechner J, Rives S, Boyer M, Bittencourt H, Bader P, Verneris MR, Stefanski HE, Myers GD, et al. Tisagenlecleucel in Children and Young Adults with B-Cell Lymphoblastic Leukemia. N Engl J Med. 2018 Feb 1;378(5):439-448
7. Maude SL, Teachey DT, Porter DL, Grupp SA. CD19-targeted chimeric antigen receptor T-cell therapy for acute lymphoblastic leukemia. Blood. 2015 Jun 25;125(26):4017-23.
8. Park JH, Rivière I, Gonen M, Wang X, Sénéchal B, Curran KJ, Sauter C, Wang Y, Santomasso B, Mead E, Roshal M, Maslak P, Davila M, Brentjens RJ, Sadelain M. Long-Term Follow-up of CD19 CAR Therapy in Acute Lymphoblastic Leukemia. N Engl J Med. 2018 Feb 1;378(5):449-459.

Checkpoint inhibition, making immunotherapy 'off-the-shelf'

While T cell therapy offers a new avenue for cancer treatment, insertion of DNA sequences encoding T cell receptor (TCR) or chimeric antigen receptor (CAR) generally requires complicated bio-techniques that involve viral vectors (retroviral, lentiviral, etc.) for gene delivery and expansion of a single cell in petri dish. Viral vectors-based genetic editing is generally a reliable and safe technique developed many decades ago and have been used in several clinical trials. However, the FDA 2006 guidance considers lentiviral and retroviral vectors to be potentially oncogenic since insertion of the vectors might happen at undesired sites of the target cell's genome. Thus, extensive and expensive biosafety tests are required before infusion of T cells. Meanwhile, expansion of engineered T cells in the culture requires a complicated complex of stimulants to preserve their cytotoxic T cell feature. This process also requires several weeks to generate adequate cell population and requires rigorous and expensive quality control. As a result, the manufacturing of clinical-grade CAR or TCR-edited T cells under good manufacturing procedure (cGMP) guidelines is an essential step and the incurring costs and complicated techniques is a bottleneck for the wide implementation of these promising therapeutic strategy.

As we mentioned, cancer cells can downregulate the cytotoxic activity of T cells via several mechanisms including modification of the surrounding microenvironment and more importantly, impose 'checkpoints' that can dampen the downstream signals of TCR and CD28 required for T cell activation. Ideally,

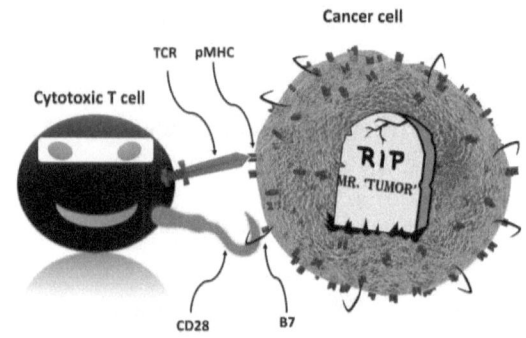

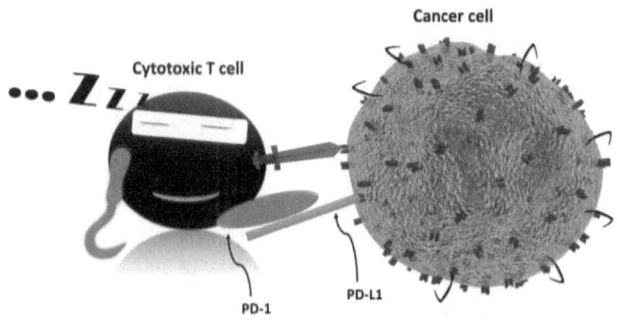

Figure 5.5: Interaction between PD-1 and PD-L1 will inhibition the binding between CD28 and B7 and thus downregulate the cytotoxic activity of T cells. Tumor cells usually have upregulated expression of PD-L1 to escape the immune surveillance.

inhibition of those checkpoints will promote T cell activation and facilitate T cell-mediated destruction of cancer cells. Theoretically, this strategy lacks tumor-specificity since all groups of T cells are promoted for activation with checkpoint inhibition. However, compared with 'living-cell' therapy based on TCR-engineered or CAR T cells, checkpoint inhibitors provide an affordable off-the-shelf immunotherapy for cancer treatment.

As we discussed, T cell activation requires activation of receptors TCR and CD28 to provide a 1st and costimulatory 2nd signals, respectively, for T cell fully activation. Meanwhile, activated T cells expresses receptors like Programmed Death 1 (PD-1) and Cytotoxic T Lymphocyte Antigen 4 (CTLA-4) that upon binding with Programmed Cell Death 1 Ligand-1 (PD-L1) and B7, respectively, can negatively regulate T cell activity. PD-1 activation can inhibit downstream pathways activated by CD28 and CD3; whereas CTLA-4 can compete with CD28 for the binding with B7. Thus, PD-1 and CTLA-4 can block both 1st and 2nd signals required for T cells fully activation. Mother Nature developed delicate positive (TCR, CD28, etc.) and negative (PD-1, CTLA-4, etc.) regulatory mechanisms to fine tune the activation status of T cell population to fight against infection while preventing generation of auto-active T cells that can cause auto-immune diseases. To prevent T cell activation, tumor cells can recruit Treg cells that have abundant CTLA-4 that have higher affinity for B 7 than CD28. As a result, not enough B 7 will be available for the binding with CD28 on T cells, blocking activation of the costimulatory signal. Meanwhile, to inhibit those activated T cells, tumor cells will overexpress PD-L1 to interact with PD-1 on T cells, leading to inhibition of signals mediated by both CD3 and CD28. By doing so, tumor cells can not only inhibit T cell activation, but also develop tolerance to fully activated T cells. Scientists outsmarted those immune evasion mechanisms of cancer cells by develop specific inhibitors that target PD-1, PD-L1 and CTLA-4 using mono-antibodies. CTL-4 inhibitors (e.g., ipilimumab), PD-1 inhibitors (e.g., Nivolumab, Pembrolizumab) and PD-L1 inhibitors (e.g., Durvalumab, Avelumab) can facilitate development and expansion of T cells with anti-tumor activities.

Since those drugs are off-the-shelf compounds, they can readily be prescribed for patients when doctors consider it suitable. Meanwhile, as normal tissue cells also depend on those checkpoint mechanisms to prevent development of auto-active T cells, side effects including skin rashes, diarrhea and hepatic toxicities, etc. associated with clinical use of checkpoint inhibitors have been reported in clinical trials. Luckily, most of these sides effects are manageable in clinic with standard care even for patients with pre-existing autoimmune disorders.

Reference

1. Monjezi R, Miskey C, Gogishvili T, Schleef M, Schmeer M, Einsele H, Ivics Z, Hudecek M. Enhanced CAR T-cell engineering using non-viral Sleeping Beauty transposition from minicircle vectors. Leukemia. 2017 Jan;31(1):186-194.
2. Levine BL, Miskin J, Wonnacott K, Keir C. Global Manufacturing of CAR T Cell Therapy. Mol Ther Methods Clin Dev. 2016 Dec 31;4:92-101.
3. Wang X, Rivière I. Clinical manufacturing of CAR T cells: foundation of a promising therapy. Mol Ther Oncolytics. 2016 Jun 15;3:16015.
4. Buchbinder EI, Desai A. CTLA-4 and PD-1 Pathways: Similarities, Differences, and Implications of Their Inhibition. Am J Clin Oncol. 2016 Feb;39(1):98-106.
5. Parry RV, Chemnitz JM, Frauwirth KA, Lanfranco

AR, Braunstein I, Kobayashi SV, Linsley PS, Thompson CB, Riley JL. CTLA-4 and PD-1 receptors inhibit T-cell activation by distinct mechanisms. Mol Cell Biol. 2005 Nov;25(21):9543-53.

6. Hsu FS, Su CH, Huang KH. A Comprehensive Review of US FDA-Approved Immune Checkpoint Inhibitors in Urothelial Carcinoma. J Immunol Res. 2017;2017:6940546.

7. Naidoo J, Page DB, Li BT, Connell LC, Schindler K, Lacouture ME, Postow MA, Wolchok JD. Toxicities of the anti-PD-1 and anti-PD-L1 immune checkpoint antibodies. Ann Oncol. 2016 Jul;27(7):1362.

8. Johnson DB, Sullivan RJ, Ott PA, Carlino MS, Khushalani NI, Ye F, Guminski A, Puzanov I, Lawrence DP, Buchbinder EI, Mudigonda T, Spencer K, Bender C, Lee J, Kaufman HL, Menzies AM, Hassel JC, Mehnert JM, Sosman JA, Long GV, Clark JI. Ipilimumab Therapy in Patients With Advanced Melanoma and Preexisting Autoimmune Disorders. JAMA Oncol. 2016 Feb;2(2):234-40.

Shuhua (Steve) Zheng, Ph.D.

Cancer vaccine, a light from future for cancer prevention

If cancer cells can be targeted for killing by cytotoxic T cells, can we use vaccines to 'educate' those immune cells so that they can readily recognize and destroy malignant cells before they progress? By doing so, we would prevent the occurrence of a specific type of tumor for whole life, similar to success we achieved using vaccines for prevention and almost eradication of chicken pox. This idea may sound unrealistic unless you know that the major causal factors of human malignancies are actually viral and/or bacterial infections. Since vaccines for virus and bacteria are relatively easy to develop and tested, we can actually prevent certain malignancies by using vaccines against those oncogenic (cancer-causing) pathogens. Based on this understanding, what we need to do next is to identify what is the major casual factor of a specific type of cancer.

For example, several members of the Human Papillomavirus (HPV) especially HPV 16 and HPV18 are identified responsible for about 70% of potentially deadly cervical cancers. Oncogenic HPVs are infectious, transmitted between persons with intimate relationships. Meanwhile, in male, more than 60% of penile cancers are caused by HPV infection and about 70% of oropharyngeal cancers may be linked to HPV infections. Consequently, FDA-approved vaccines for HPVs will serve the purpose of preventing HPV infection and by doing so, lowering the possibility of having cervical, penile and oropharyngeal cancers. Meanwhile, studies showed that hepatitis B virus (HBV) and hepatitis C virus (HCV) infection is a one major risk factor for people to develop deadly liver cancer. Consequently, another major benefit in vaccinations against HBV and HCV is lowering the possibility of having liver cancer. Please refer to CDC (Centers for Disease Control and Prevention) for updated recommendations on HPV, HBV and HCV vaccinations. Besides viruses, some chronic bacterial infections are also identified as major contributing oncogenic factor. For example, the bacterial Helicobacter pylori (H. pylori) was well established the major cause of gastric cancer (stomach cancer), the second leading cause of cancer-related deaths worldwide. While bacterial infections are relatively easier to clear out compared with viral infections, H. pylori infection are sometimes difficult to treat especially with the development of resistant strains. H. pylori is mainly acquired during childhood and may persist throughout life if untreated. While vaccines for H. pylori are still under development, close monitoring and timely treatment for infected patients will be beneficial for prevention of gastric cancer.

Are there any ways to use vaccines to benefit the treatment of cancer that are not caused by viral or bacterial infections? Studies in this field are now generally focusing on developing the so-called therapeutic cancer vaccines, which use the vaccines to treat the cancer instead of preventing its occurrence as typical vaccines will do. Strategies involved are based on the general idea we already learnt from T cell based therapies. For example, cancer cells derived from the cancer patients can be engineered to express B7 molecules and then reintroduced back into the patient by infusion. Those engineered tumor cells can act like vaccines since they are now more likely to guide T cells develop anti-tumor specificity. Also, antigen presenting cells (APCs) (a group of cells that are mainly responsible for presentation of

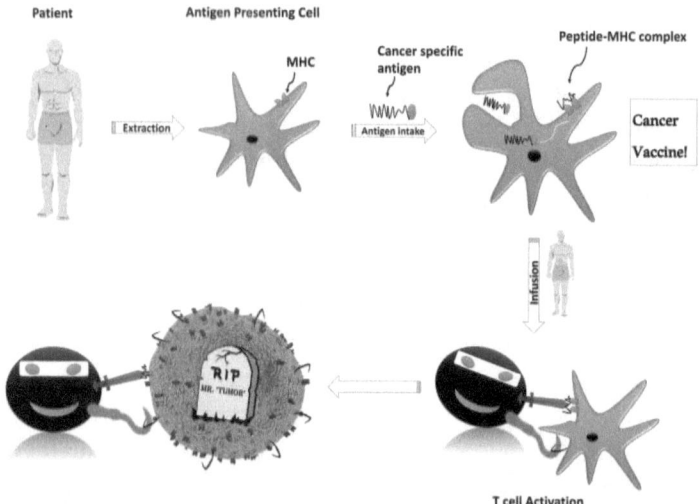

Figure 5.6: The generation of tumor vaccines are quite a complicated process. Briefly, the antigen presenting cells (APCs) derived from the patient are cultured with tumor specific antigen. APCs will engulf the antigens and present in on cell surface by MHCs, generating peptide-MHC complex. These engineered APCs will be introduced back into the patient to stimulate the generation of T cells with specificity against the antigen. Those cytotoxic T cells will then attack tumor cells.

antigen to naïve T cells via peptide-MHC complex to stimulate antigen-specific T cell activation) derived from the cancer patients can be treated with cancer specific antigens. Then the reinfused APCs will educate the naive T cells to develop T cell receptors with anti-tumor specificity. Sipuleucel-T is so far the only FDA approved cancer vaccine that were developed based on this strategy. It is mainly used for the treatment of prostate cancer that are resistant to traditional therapies. Briefly, APCs derived for the prostate cancer patients will be presented with a fusion protein that includes a prostate antigen called prostatic acid phosphatase (PAP). The APCs will engulfed the PAP, process it and present the PAP-derived peptide on cell surface using MHCs. These APC cells are re-introduced back into the patient via infusion. Then, those APCs will induce the development of cytotoxic T cells that can recognize this prostate antigen, facilitating the destruction of cancer cells. Currently, the costs of using Sipuleucel-T for prostate cancer treatment is not cheap. However, with the great success of the APC-based cancer vaccine, we will see more successful stories and companies will be encouraged to develop more financially competitive treatment plans.

Reference

1. Maver PJ, Poljak M. Progress in prophylactic human papillomavirus (HPV) vaccination in 2016: A literature review. Vaccine. 2017 Aug 8. pii: S0264-410X(17)31064-2.
2. Di Bisceglie AM. Hepatitis B and hepatocellular carcinoma. Hepatology. 2009 May;49(5 Suppl):S56-60.
3. Sokic-Milutinovic A, Alempijevic T, Milosavljevic T. Role of Helicobacter pylori infection in gastric carcinogenesis: Current knowledge and future directions. World J Gastroenterol. 2015 Nov 7;21(41):11654-72.
4. Talebi Bezmin Abadi A. Vaccine against Helicobacter pylori: Inevitable approach.
5. Sutton P, Boag JM. Status of vaccine research and development for Helicobacter py World J Gastroenterol. 2016 Mar 21;22(11):3150-7. lori. Vaccine. 2018 Apr 4. pii: S0264-410X(18)30017-3.
6. Kantoff PW, Higano CS, Shore ND, Berger ER, Small

EJ, Penson DF, Redfern CH, Ferrari AC, Dreicer R, Sims RB, Xu Y, Frohlich MW, Schellhammer PF; IMPACT Study Investigators. Sipuleucel-T immunotherapy for castration-resistant prostate cancer. N Engl J Med. 2010 Jul 29;363(5):411-22.
7. Guo C, Manjili MH, Subjeck JR, Sarkar D, Fisher PB, Wang XY. Therapeutic cancer vaccines: past, present, and future. Adv Cancer Res. 2013;119:421-75.